Transfusion of Blood Preserved by Freezing

SAJIO SUMIDA, M.D.

Chief, Division of Cardiovascular Surgery
and Medical Low Temperature Unit
The National Fukuoka Central Hospital, Fukuoka, Japan

IGAKU SHOIN LTD. TOKYO

J. B. LIPPINCOTT COMPANY
PHILADELPHIA AND TORONTO

Sole Distributor in the United States and Canada
J. B. LIPPINCOTT COMPANY, East Washington Square, Philadelphia Pa., U.S.A.

ISBN 0-397-58132-7

Library of Congress Catalog Card Number: 73-14029

Printed and bound in Japan

Foreword

During the past ten years there have been significant advances in the field of blood transfusion. Clinical problems associated with blood and blood transfusions nonetheless remain acute in several aspects. In his monograph Dr. SUMIDA has elucidated many of these complex problems, as well as he has given voice to various means of attempting to solve these crucial problems.

One of the most significant advances in the area of blood transfusion has been a greater understanding of the basic mechanisms of freezing and freezing injury. This understanding has gone hand in hand with, and has been partially necessitated by, the worldwide movement from what was once primarily a paid donor population to a system that now is supported mostly by volunteer blood donors. Traditional problems of maintaining adequate blood bank inventories have been somewhat aggravated by this move from paid to volunteer donors, however, and the ability to preserve blood by freezing has played a vital role in dealing effectively with the clinical problem of assuring availibility of high quality blood at all times.

Another major benefit that derived from an increased use of frozen blood is a lowering of the incidence of serum hepatitis resulting from transfusions. Serum hepatitis has long been recognized as one of the foremost hazards associated with blood transfusions, and the success we have seen with hepatitis through the use of frozen blood is a strong stimulus in encouraging further research and application in the area of frozen blood.

I personally am very pleased that many of my previous co-workers, Dr. TSUYOSHI MIURA, Dr. SHINJI YUASA, Dr. SHICHISABURO ABO, and Dr. HIROSHI SUZUKI, have joined with Dr. SAJIO SUMIDA, and my many other Japanese friends, to advance the use of frozen blood in Japan. Their expanding efforts have made a notable contribution both to basic research and to clinical awareness of the benefits of frozen blood throughout the world.

CHARLES E. HUGGINS

Foreword

The biological effects of cold have been observed for centuries. But the relationship between low temperature and life remained largely unexplained until 1940, when LUYET and GEHENIO published their classic treatise, "Life and Death at Low Temperatures." Since that time, increasing numbers of researchers from various disciplines have become attracted to the new and rapidly expanding field of *Cryobiology*. The observation in 1951 by AUDREY SMITH that glycerol protects red cells from the lethal effects of freezing opened new vistas for the long-term preservation of the cellular components of blood by means of freezing and thawing.

The introduction of new therapeutic medical procedures has created an ever increasing demand not only for whole blood but also for its components: erythrocytes, leukocytes, and platelets. This clinical application has been a major driving force for the vast amount of research into the methods of preserving red cells and platelets for use in transfusion.

In this monograph, Dr. SUMIDA explains freezing damage to red cells in terms of his own observations with a cryomicroscope. This is then followed by a comprehensive summary of author's *in vitro* and *in vivo* clinical studies on frozen blood, using both the "high glycerol-slow freeze" and "low glycerol-rapid freeze" methods of preserving red cells. The monograph is not restricted to the preservation of red cells, but also encompasses platelet preservation. The author presents a promising approach to the freezing of platelets. As this method becomes more practical, it will enable the increased use of frozen platelet preparations for the treatment of idiopathic and iatrogenic thrombocytopenias.

Frozen blood *per se* must prove itself effective, regardless of the method of freezing. New technological advances in containers and methods of post-thaw processing of frozen blood have renewed interest in it. Frozen blood is now coming into its own as a practical reality rather than as an esoteric commodity. The obvious advantage of having both rare and common bloods readily accessible has recently been overshadowed by the observation that frozen blood is also associated with the decreased presence of potentially immunizing histocompatibility antigens and a lowered incidence in transfusion hepatitis. The improved patient care realized with frozen blood more than justifies its slightly increased cost. Frozen blood implies features of purity, potency, and safety not obtainable in liquid stored blood, and still remains the only hope for indefinite storage. It is therefore only a matter of time before frozen blood will become an integral part of every blood bank in supplementing the supply of fresh blood.

The interest and enthusiasm for the successful freezing of red cells and platelets in Japan are exemplified in this very elegant monograph. Without doubt it will serve as a valuable reference source and do much to educate students, stimulate researchers, and promote more widespread use of frozen red cells and platelets.

The New York Blood Center
March, 1973

ARTHUR W. ROWE

Preface

"Frozen Blood Transfusion" is a new technique of transfusion appeared in the last half of 20th century. The first successful transfusion of frozen red cells was done by P. L. MOLLISON and H. A. SLOVITER in 1951. After that this transfusion bloomed in the United States of America during the Vietnam Conflict. In 1965, this medical art was introduced to Japan by C. E. HUGGINS. He demonstrated us the unique procedure to wash out glycerol by the agglomeration phenomenon at the 13th Annual Meeting of Japan Society for Blood Transfusion in 1965. We were deeply impressed with his lecture, and an idea of the realization of this epoch-making technique in Japan occurred to me in a moment. However, it took unexpectedly a long way to actualize the dream. From the practical point of view, no detailed explanation has been made in HUGGINS' papers, and our failures repeated.

Hemoglobinuria was one of the most hazardous complications. Several modifications were needed to subside those side effects. As the volume of blood collection is 200 ml in Japan and 400 ml in the United States, so we had to design all over again; the blood freezing container, centrifuge and cytoglomerator. "Seeing is believing." In order to understand concretely the blood freezing practices and the fundamental problems, I visited the Frozen Blood Section (Chief, C. E. HUGGINS) in Massachusetts General Hospital in Boston in 1966, and to the Laboratory of Cryobiology (Chief, A. W. ROWE) in the New York Blood Center in New York in 1968, and the Institute of Low Temperature Science of Hokkaido University (Professor, T. NEI). In this way, I have been interested in the frozen blood over the past eight years. Especially I have done the best of my ability to master the practices of freezing and thawing of blood cells, so I emphasized the practical aspects of blood freezing process in this short monograph, including the results of laboratory and clinical studies made by myself at the Toho University Hospital in Tokyo and the National Fukuoka Central Hospital in Fukuoka.

I payed my effort to describe the original data differ from those of other researchers as much as possible. For these reasons, I spared the statements about the freeze-preservation of bone marrow and leukocytes in the present book, although these cells are processed in a routine in our Frozen Blood Unit. I tried in detail to mention the procedures of freeze-preservation of red blood cells and platelets, and to persent the full informations of practical support at the frozen blood transfusion. Countermeasures considering the side effects: serum hepatitis and hemoglobinuria are taken.

Recently, new methods are developed one after the other and they are utilized by each blood center in the world. However, no single method appears to be satisfactory for the frozen blood processing of the individual cell types.

I do believe that the frozen blood processed by the techniques introduced in the present book will widely used by the public.

"All scientific progress is progress in method." It is my hope that this monograph will aid in the processing of the freeze-preservation of blood cells and stimulate further interest in the development of newer and more effective techniques for the frozen blood transfusion.

March 1, 1973

SAJIO SUMIDA

Acknowledgements

I am deeply indebted to Dr. C. E. HUGGINS and Dr. A. W. ROWE who not only assisted in the realization of frozen blood transfusion in Japan, but also revised, proofread and corrected the manuscript of this book. Without their international cooperations, this work would not be completed. And, I am especially honored to have had the forewords written by them to this short monograph.

I am most grateful for the frequent suggestions, stimulating informations and helpful discussions with Professor T. NEI and Dr. T. MIURA. Professor T. NEI sent me several copies of very rare references. I also want to thank Professor B. J. LUYET for permission to quote his expressions of the cryomicroscopic observation. Several words having quotation-marks were cited from his papers already published elsewhere.

I should like to thank Professor S. MINAKAMI for his courtesies in specific inquiries and for providing his file of recondite references to literature on red cells metabolism.

I am much indebted to Professor K. INOKUCHI, Dr. H. KOGA and Dr. T. TASHIRO who gave me the opportunity and place for resuming the research of the frozen blood transfusion in Fukuoka City. Dr. H. KOGA, Director of the National Fukuoka Central Hospital sponsored our Frozen Blood Section and Medical Low Temperature Unit.

I also want to thank Dr. M. YOSHINARI and Dr. J. YASUDA for their continuing guidances and excellent suggestions on the fundamental and technical problems in the hematology and blood transfusion.

I particularly want to acknowledge the invaluable help of my secretary Miss Y. JOUJIMA, Phar. B. and my collaborators, who have been responsible for the technical assistance and processed about 4,000 units of frozen bloods that contributed to the progress of this work.

This research was supported by Grants from the Ministry of Welfare and the National Institute of Health (Japan).

Finally, I want to thank my publisher, Igaku Shoin Ltd. for present courtesy.

The Author

Contents

1

Introduction

Citrate-Dextrose (CD) blood originated from ROUS and TURNER (1916) was transfused to save the lives of many battle casualties during World War I. Between 1914 and 1918 the techniques of blood transfusion were remarkably simplified. SHIODA, H. (Professor of Tokyo University), who had been in Europe as a Chief of Relief Party of Japan Red Cross, observed the actual circumstances of blood transfusion in the battle field. SHIODA started the research of blood transfusion as soon as he came back to Japan, and 200 ml of CD blood was transfused into a patient with heavy anemia from uterine myoma on February 28, 1919. It was 18 years after the vital discovery of the ABO blood groups made by KARL LANDSTEINER (1900). After that, GOTO, S. (Professor of Kyushu University, Fukuoka) also succeeded the blood transfusion of CD blood for a postoperative patient of chronic pyothorax on the April of 1919.

Blood transfusion was definitely popularized in Japan on November 5, 1930, when HAMAGUCHI, O., the Primeminister of Japan, who was shot by an assassin, escaped death by a transfusion of blood donated by his son with filial affection and the news was spread by newspapers all over Japan. It was just the year that the Father of Immunohematology received the Nobel prise in medicine for his discovery of the ABO blood groups.

Acid-Citrate-Dextrose (ACD) blood appeared during World War II (1939–1949) also saved lives of casualties. Taking this opportunity banks for keeping blood at $+5°C$ had been established in Russia, the U.S.A. and England. STRUMIA (1940) and GREAVES (1946) found freeze-dried plasma, which could be kept without deteriorating for months or years at atmospheric temperature. As a plasma expander, REPPE (1940) discovered PVP, GRÄNWALL and INGELMAN (1944) dextran, and TOMODA and INOKUCHI (1944) arginic acid.

The Korean Conflict (1950–1953) outbroke and the ACD blood and freeze-dried plasma played important roles in combat zones. The War came to an end, leaving a serious and often fatal complication "serum hepatitis" of blood transfusion.

By 1950, 50 or more blood banks were established in Japan. They began to supply ACD blood and plasma, and the table was spread for serum hepatitis at the same time. The safe period of storage of blood was, however, limited to 3 weeks at $+4°C$.

LUYET (1949) cooled thin films of blood at an ultra-rapid rate in liquid nitrogen for indefinite periods at that temperature without deteriorating. This method was of academic interest, but did not seem applicable to banking of blood on a large scale (MERYMAN, 1957). New possibilities were opened up by the demonstration that glycerol protected avian spermatozoa against the otherwise damaging effects of freezing to,

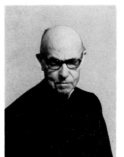 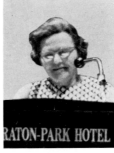 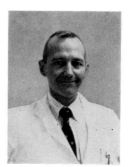

LUYET, B.   SMITH, A. U.   HUGGINS, C. E.

storage at, and thawing from very low temperature. This led indirectly to resume
work on freezing red blood cells (SMITH, 1961). AUDREY U. SMITH (1950) at the National
Institute for Medical Research found that red blood cells could also be preserved in
media containing glycerol in the frozen state. When they were frozen to and thawed
from −20°C, −40°C or −79°C in presence of 10% or 15% glycerol the great majority
of the cells were intact, whereas erythrocytes suspended in media free from glycerol
were completely hemolysed by freezing and thawing in the same way (SMITH, 1950).
The first patient with chronic leukaemia received 100 ml of a suspension of the previously frozen erythrocytes. No unfavourable reactions were noticed (MOLLISON and
SLOVITER, 1951). As a result frozen red cells could not be widely used for transfusion.
TULLIS (1956) freeze-preserved red blood cells by use of SMITH's procedures and succeeded the first transfusion of frozen blood after washing out glycerol after thawing by
COHN's fractionator. TULLIS also found that frozen red cell transfusion had neither
transfusion reaction nor serum hepatitis, however COHN's fractionator was too complicated to be popularized.

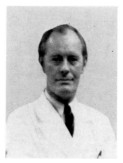 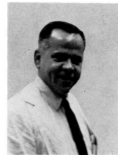 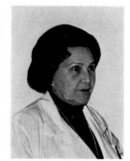

KRIJNEN, H. W.   ROWE, A. W.   VINOGRAD-FINKEL, F. R.

In 1963, CHARLES E. HUGGINS evolved a unique technique to remove glycerol at Massachusetts General Hospital. The key to the HUGGINS' method is in the washing of
the red cells, which enables them to separate from the glycerol by "clumping". Every
physician and nurse has witnessed the clumping of red cells that takes place within the
syring of intravenous injection of glucose in water. He applied this phenomenon to de-
glycerolize from red cells and named "reversible agglomeration". His method to wash
out glycerol was widely accepted not only in the U.S.A. but also in the foreign coun-

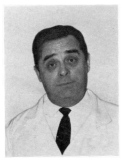 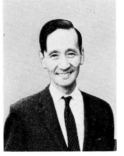 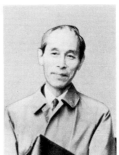

KISSELEV, A. E.   ASAHINA, E.   NEI, T.

tries. Recently, the Vietnam Conflict and civilian experience have emphasized the improtance of preservation and transfusion of blood. A frozen blood bank system increased the *capability* and *flexibility* of the standard blood bank system in treating a wide variety of surgical and medical conditions in war and peace. HUGGINS, C. E. visited Japan as a invited speaker at the 13th Annual Meeting for Japan Society for Blood Transfusion (Professor HAYASHI, S., President) and gave an epoch-making lec-

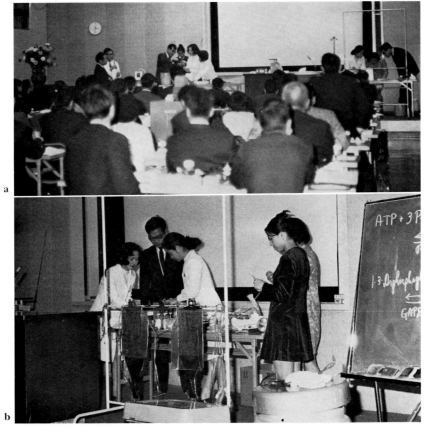

Fig. 1 The first lecture course concerning frozen blood practice was held at the National Fukuoka Central Hospital on January 21–22, 1971 (*upper*), the second on January 20–22, 1972 (*lower*), and the third on January 25–26, 1973.

ture of "Frozen Blood". This was the fuse which set ablaze frozen blood transfusion in Japan.

Inspired by HUGGINS' lecture previously mentioned, the first transfusion of frozen blood was done by SUMIDA (1966) on the October of 1965 at the Toho University (Tokyo). After that SUMIDA moved from Tokyo to Fukuoka, where the frozen blood center was firstly set up in 1969. The first course concerning frozen blood and the practical procedures was held on January 21–22, 1971, and the second was on January 20–21, 1972 at the National Fukuoka Central Hospital (Fig. 1). One hundred and fifty attendants gathered from 100 facilities all over Japan, and they heard epoch-making lectures on the fundamental and practical problems of frozen blood and saw the demonstrations of frozen blood processing. Since the beginning of the frozen blood center, about 3000 units of frozen blood were supplied for 400 patients. And, frozen blood constitutes about 30% of the total units of blood transfusion in our hospital.

2

Erythrocyte

CRYOMICROSCOPIC OBSERVATION OF FREEZING AND THAWING PROCESS IN RED CELLS

Object

It has been the most basic research to observe the freeze-thaw process of red cells by light microscope, because anatomy of the freezing process in biological materials by light microscopy has offered a very effective means for resolving the mechanism of freezing injury. Therefore, it might be hardly necessary to review here again previous research at the light microscopic level. Especially, LUYET's observations (1965) were complete, and there will be no original findings in this monograph. Although several theories have been proposed to explain irreversible freezing damage, all of them agree that the mechanisms of ice formation play a major role, as mentioned by DILLER (1970).

There have been two different types of ice formation observed in cell suspension. Ice crystals are formed only extracellularly at relatively low cooling rates resulting in salt injury emphasized by LOVELOCK (1953), and they are formed both intracellularly and extracellularly at relatively high cooling rates resulting in mechanical injury proposed by NEI (1962) and confirmed by SUMIDA (1971). The magnitude of the governing cooling rate and its effect are dependent upon many parameters, the more important of which are the species of cell being frozen and whether a cryoprotective agent has been added to the specimen (DILLER et al., 1970). However, it is interesting to note that in the case of both freezing and thawing process, hypothesis regarding injury mechanisms are formed on the basis of observations made on the specimen prior to and subsequent to, but never during, these processes. There is no information about the dynamics of these processes. On the basis of such limited information, conflicts and contradictions exist among the various investigators regarding the mechanisms of injury (DILLER et al., 1970). Light microscopy offered a very effective means for resolving these differences, but it was difficult to settle this problem to the satisfaction of all. Because from the clinical point of view in the frozen red cells, it was satisfactory in determining hematocrit and supernatant hemoglobin concentration of red cell suspensions after freeze-thaw processes. Strictly speaking, the recovery rate and the viability of freeze-preserved living cells are more important in clinical medicine than the resolution of injury mechanisms. Therefore, we think the cryomicroscopic observation may be, in the true sense of the word, a scientific interest.

SMITH (1951), LUYET (1965), NEI (1967) and RINFRET (1968) have used this method previously and reported many beautiful photographs but their tests covered only a small range of temperatures and cooling rates. DILLER (1970) pointed out that these limitations were due, in part, to the difficulties associated with the control of the heat transfer rates and with the instrumentation of the specimen to obtain accurate measurements of rapidly changing temperatures. In spite of these limitations, the results of these early experiments are impressive and indicate that more extensive optical studies are warranted.

Design

The specific design of the thermodynamic system is shown schematically in Figs. 2, 3, and 4. The refrigeration chamber, 80 mm in diameter, is made of special heatproof materials. Inside the chamber, the cold end (center) and the hot end (center left) are located. A 22 mm specimen glass bridges the two ends and is fastened with clamps. The specimen to be viewed can be directly mounted on the specimen glass and then covered with a cover slip of the approximate thickness. The red blood cells suspended in various media can be observed with a phase contrast dry objective. With this objective, maximum useful total magnification is limited by resolution considerations to approximately × 800. The viewing end of the microscope is fitted with a camera such as a 35 mm for static studies or a 16 mm motionpicture camera for dynamic studies. The Bolex camera was used for slow speed work, 12 to 64 exposures per second.

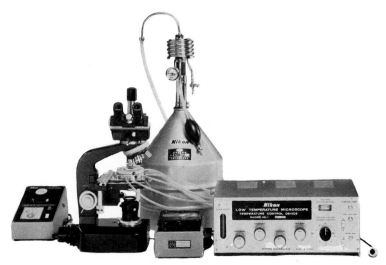

Fig. 2   Photograph of the cryomicroscope, and the elements of the equipment.
Refrigerant supplier: A container with the freeze material, nitrogen, and an automatic device attached.
Refrigeration chamber: The chamber in which specimens are frozen.
Control box: The paneled box for the control of different low temperatures generation.
Precision thermometer: A thermistor thermometer.
Silicone rubber tubes and electrical cords for connecting the above units.

The position of the thermistor is about 3 mm from the cold end, the thermistor is parallel to the end. When the equipment is used for measuring freezing points, no cover glass on the specimen is preferred, so that more precise temperature information

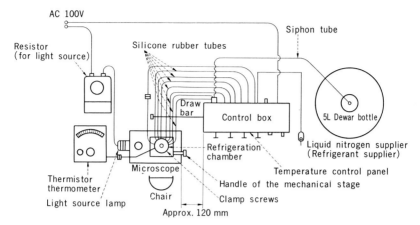

Fig. 3 Arrangement and connection of the elements.

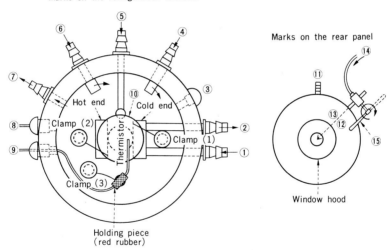

Fig. 4 Freezing chamber of cryomicroscope.

The marked parts are as follows:
1. Inlet for liquid nitrogen. } (used in gradient refrigeration)
2. Outlet for liquid nitrogen.
3. Spare hole.
4. Inlet for low-temperature (0– –120°C) gas (used in clearing or circumstance refrigeration).
5. Inlet for the lower defogging curtain gas.
6. Inlet for high-temperature (0– +60°C) gas (used at circumstance thawing or heating).
7. Outlet for exhaust gas.
8. Heater terminal (used in gradient thawing).
9. Thermistor.
10. Sample holder.
11. Inlet for the upper defogging curtain gas.
12, 13, 14. Inlet for liquid nitrogen used for instantaneous rapid cooling.
15. Liquid nitrogen injection nozzle (used with three-way valve).

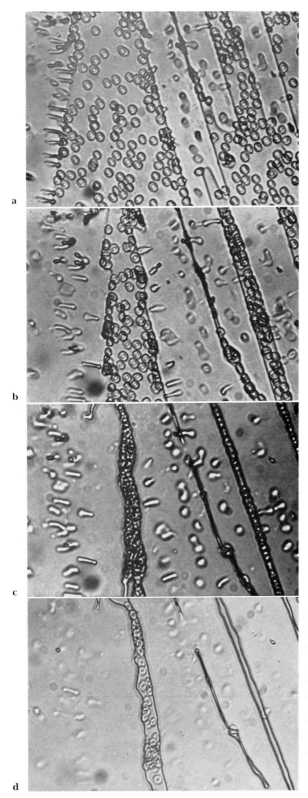

Fig. 5 Changes observed at the same field when a film of blood in a 0.9% saline without any additives, frozen at −5°C and then cooled at the rate of 30–40°C per minute to −80°C and gradually rewarmed at the same rate above 0°C. *Magnification:* ×400.

a: Film in the frozen state at −70°C.

f and g: Films during rewarming. There remains no red cell in the channels of thawed medium (h).

These figures show that hemolysis is mainly caused during the freezing process were the red cells frozen by the upper-

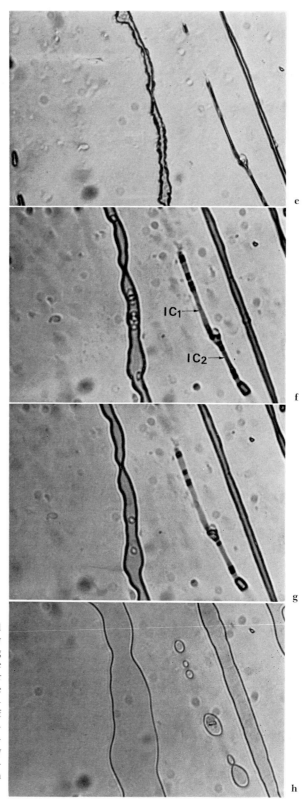

given conditions. The cells are squeezed between ice columns through remarkably narrow channels where the suspending medium is being concentrated, and the others are compressed and streched under ice column. "Plasmolysis" or shrinkage are seen in Fig. 5-e, f, and g, which are resulted from an endosmotic penetration of water into the cells when the solute concentration of unfrozen medium is decreased by the melting of the ice immediately surrounding the cells. Some of ice channels (IC_1 and IC_2) fused to be buried in the ice block.

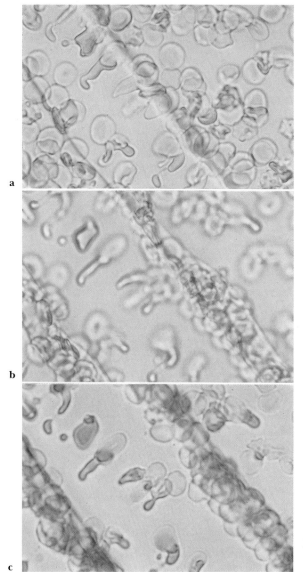

a

b

c

Fig. 6   Figs. a, b, c show mechanical hemolysis under and between ice columns at the temperature of 10°C. *Magnification*:   ×800.

can be obtained and the thermistor into direct contact with the specimen.   However, the specimen is so thin (about 10–20 μ) that the actual temperature difference across the specimen is essencially zero.   It is not possible to measure intracellular temperature gradient with this system.   When the window hood is installed on the refrigera-

Fig. 7   "Deplasmolysis" resulting in hemolysis during thawing process from −20°C to the near-zero temperature. *Magnification*:   ×800.
When the temperature rise, the channels containing unfrozen medium and red cells gradually and remarkably increase in size.   They begin to swell or deplasmolyze and lose their crenation.   With further melting of the ice and further dilution of unfrozen plasma, deplasmolysis continues and the cells seem to regain their normal shape, sizes and appearance.   Then, as the last vestiges of ice melt away, the cells hemolyze and fade from view.   The same findings are seen in Fig. 5.

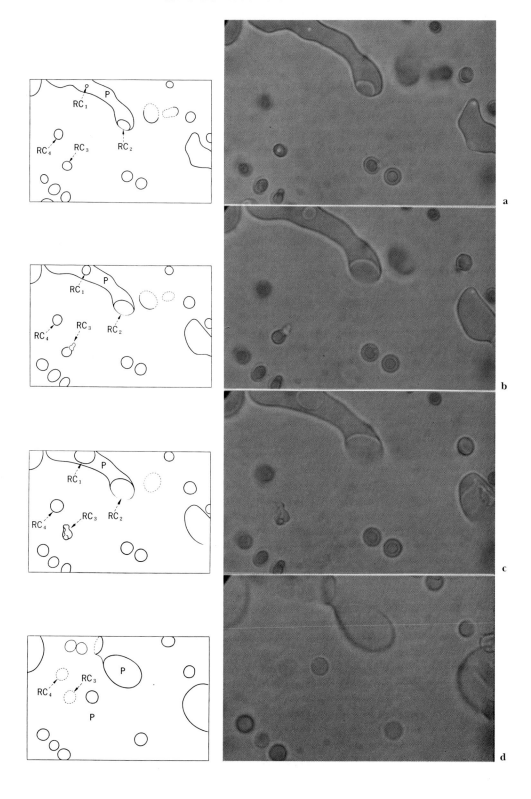

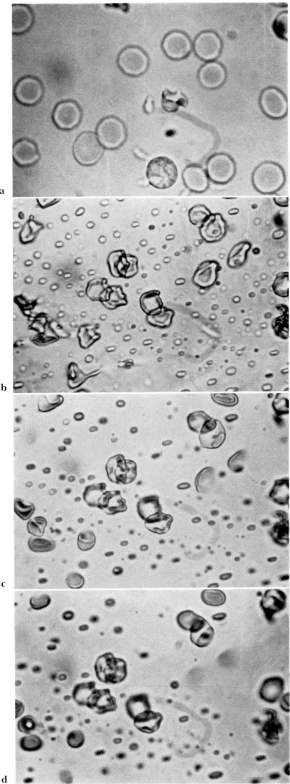

a

b

c

d

Fig. 8   Changes observed in a film of
blood frozen at about −110°C by the highly instantaneous cooling and thawed by
the circumstance rewarming.
a : Red cells and a white cell are suspended in a plasma-0.9% saline medium
without any additives.
b : Film in the frozen state at −120°C.
The cells, still buried in the ice blocks,
assume different shape, decrease in volume,
show hemolysis.
c–g : Same area as in Fig. 8-b after rewarming to −10°C, −8°C, −7°C, −5°C,
−4°C, and −3°C, respectively. As the
temperature raised, the pools of unfrozen
medium, of which some one entrap the
red cells, widen and coalesce. During
this process there is generally hemolysis
in succession.
h : A completely thawed preparation.
Several faded red cells and a white cell

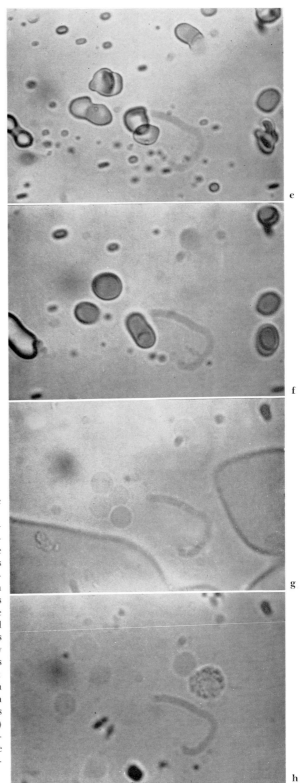

are seen. Usually leukocytes never lose their identity.

RAPATZ et al. (1966) showed the following features by electronmicroscopic observations of sections of frozen bovine leukocytes and platelets: (1) the cells contain numerous intracellular and intranuclear ice cavities; (2) the cavities in the nucleus are generally larger and less numerous and the partitions between the cavities are thicker than in the central regions of the nucleus; (3) the cavities in the nuclei of leukocyte are considerably smaller than those in the erythrocytes occasionally present in a preparation; (4) the plasma contains ice cavities which are enormous in comparison to those in the cells; (5) in suspnsion of leukocytes frozen slowly (at a rate of 1°C per minute) there is no evidence of intracellular freezing; (6) platelets show also crystalline formations similar to those in the leukocytes.

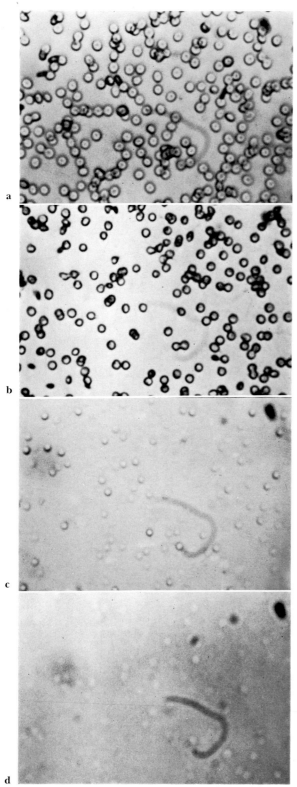

Fig. 9   The highly instantaneous freezing and thawing. Film of red cells suspension in 0.9% saline frozen at the rate of about 100–150°C per second to −120°C and immediately rewarmed at the rate of about 100°C per second. *Magnification*: ×400.

a: Area shown in the frozen state at −120°C. Red cells are buried in the ice blocks. No hemolysis is seen.

b: Same area during instantaneous rewarming and thawing. The ice blocks start to melt. The cells within the pools of thawed medium are considered to be injured. About half numbers of cells already lose their identity.

c and **d:** When the temperature raise instantaneously in 2–3 seconds, many cells appear to survive the freeze-thaw cycle, however they are still vague in each small pool of thawed medium. Such cells become more vague in contour gradually and fade out in 10–20 seconds in the completely thawed medium. These evidences suggest that the red cells are irreversibly injured at the process of freezing. We assume that hemolysis in the true sense of the word occurs during the process of freezing, and the cell membranes lost their semipermiability by the instantaneous freezing. LUYET and PRIBOR (1965) have assumed that hemolysis was actually seen to take place during thawing, however the irreparable damage might have been caused in the course of the initial freezing. Electronmicroscope photographs revealed the rapid freezing of whole blood resulted in the formation of intracellular ice in almost all the cells (RAPATZ and LUYET, 1963).

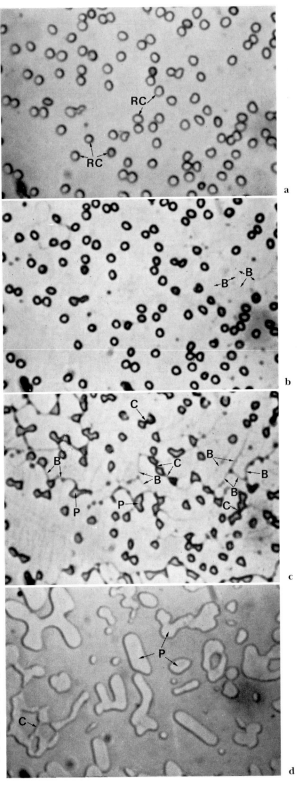

Fig. 10   A film of blood suspension in a plasma-0.9% saline medium, frozen at −120°C by the instantaneous cooling and thawed to −3°C by the circumstance rewarming, which is rather slower than the instantaneous rewarming.

a: Film in the frozen state at −100°C. The cells are trapped within the pools with highly concentrated medium.

b–d: Film during rewarming.   B, borderlines between arborescent units in frozen plasma ; C, channels of concentrated thawed plasma ; RC, red cells in the pools of melted and concentrated medium ; P, pools of melted fluid. *Magnification* :   ×400.

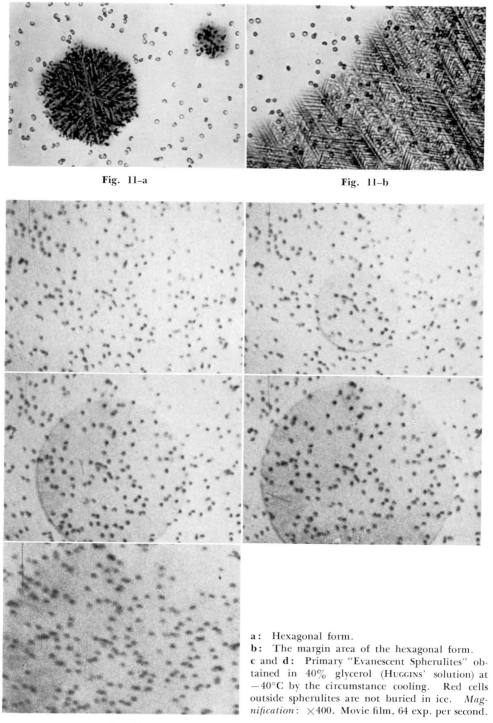

Fig. 11-a

Fig. 11-b

Fig. 11-c

a : Hexagonal form.
b : The margin area of the hexagonal form.
c and d : Primary "Evanescent Spherulites" obtained in 40% glycerol (HUGGINS' solution) at —40°C by the circumstance cooling. Red cells outside spherulites are not buried in ice. *Magnification*: ×400. Movie film, 64 exp. per second.

Fig. 11   The principal types of ice crystallization units obtained when glycerol solution of 40% are frozen at various rates.

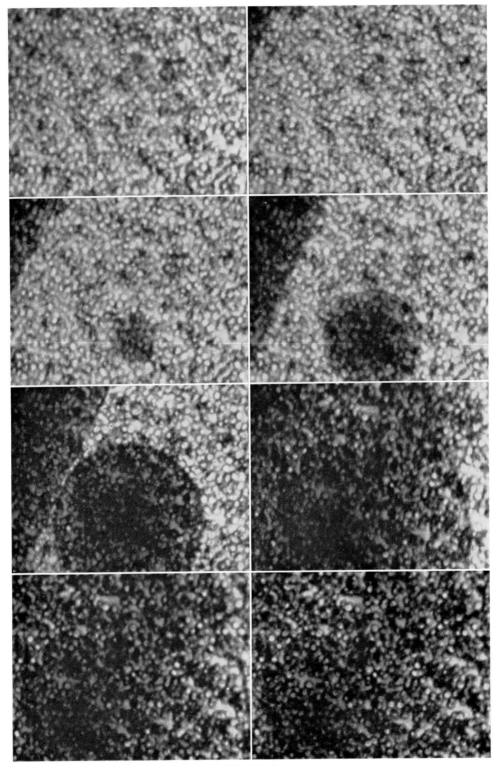

Fig. 11–d

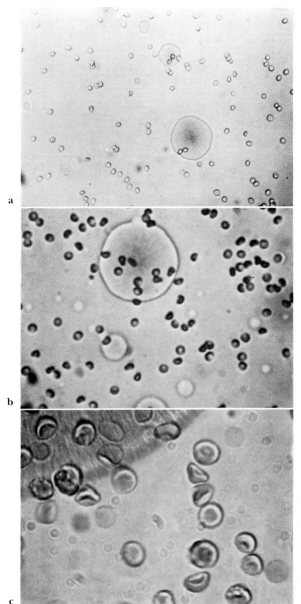

a

b

c

Fig. 12   A film of blood in 40% glycerol (Huggins' solution) primarily frozen
at −40°C by the circumstance rapid cooling, and then cooled more rapidly to
−60°C or lower.
a and **b**: "Secondary Evanescent Spherulites" were formed on the primary crystallization.   Red cells outside spherulites
are buried in an aqueous solution in the
"amorphous state" or in the "vitrification".
Magnification :   ×400.

tion chamber lid in the prescribed position, the chamber is completely sealed thereby
providing a stable inside temperature condition.   In this case, however, the objective
of the microscope must have a long focusing length.   If high magnification is required,
the window hood must be removed to bring the objective close to the specimen.   Even
in the latter case, clouding of the lenses will never occur owing to the gas curtains.
Injection nozzles are used in instantaneous rapid cooling and instantaneous thawing.
The liquid nitrogen is injected through the nozzle into the chamber directly onto the
specimen, which is cooled instantaneously to −120°C or lower in 1–2 seconds.   The
operation of the high-temperature nozzle is similar to the above.   After the above pre-

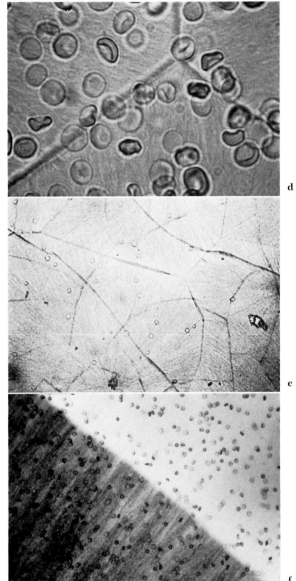

c and d: "Coase spherulites" formed in
40% glycerol (Huggins' solution). Smooth
surfaced red cells can be identified in the
ice plates at −80°C. "Borderlines between
arborescent units" in frozen medium are
distinguishable in Fig. 12-d. *Magnification*: ×800.
e and f: "Primary Evanescent Spherulites" developed from the cool end. Crack
formations are seen in Fig. 12-e. *Magnification*: ×200.

paratory operations, the respective procedures for each purpose are proceeded: (a) the
gradient cooling, (b) the circumstance cooling, and (c) the highly instantaneous cooling, and the rewarming is possible respectively.

Changes occurring during the rewarming and freezing of red cell suspension in 0.9% saline at −80°C

The film of fresh human blood, collected in ACD solution and diluted 2–3 times
with 0.9% saline, was thin enough to form a single layer of cells, which was frozen in
the refrigeration chamber of the cryomicroscope followed cooling at a cooling rate of

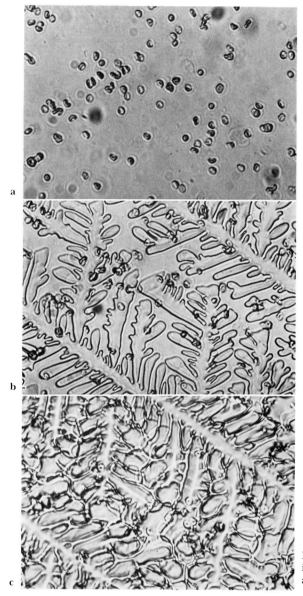

Fig. 13   Film of red cells suspended in 39% glycerol (HUGGINS' solution) frozen at −35°C to −45°C and then cooled to

1–3000°C per minute near to −80 – −120°C. The freezing was initiated at the cold end and developed to the hot end by gradient cooling. And, the freezing developed irregular or diffuse by circumstance or highly instantaneous cooling. Specimens frozen at −80°C or −120°C were kept at that temperature for several minutes and then re-warmed at the rate of about 30°C per minute to 0°C or more. The course of events during freezing and thawing was observed or photographed in still or motion pictures. In the slow freezing (at −5°C and −10°C) several minutes was allowed for the development in the plasma-saline mixture, of ice boards with heavy thickness as shown in Figs. 5, 6, and 7. In the rapid freezing, the ice crystals were so fine as to be practically indistinguishable, and the field of frozen medium had a smooth or finely granular

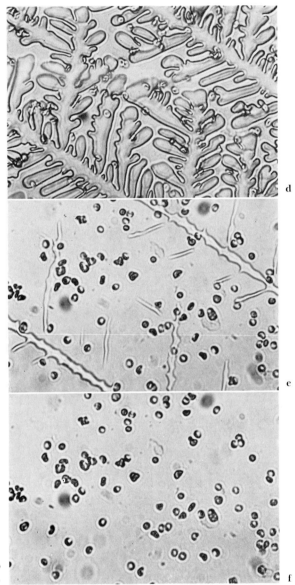

d

e

−80°C or lower and rewarmed. No
hemolysis occurred. *Magnification*: ×400.

f

appearance as shown in Fig. 8. The red blood cells in 0.9% saline were totally hemolyzed during the cooling process at a cooling rate of 1–10°C per minute, and at the
temperature ranging from the freezing point to −80°C, although it had also been
known that the temperature-time history during the thawing process played an important part in determining the final condition of the red cells. Some red cells remained
unhemolyzed when they had been in the frozen state for just a few seconds. Two pat-
terns of hemolysis resulting from mechanical and salt injury were noted as already suggested by previous investigators (LUYET 1965, LOVELOCK 1953, and NEI 1967). Red
cells in 0.9% saline became deformed, compressed by the ice column from both sides (at
the ice channel) resulting in crenation and increased osmotic pressure. Finally hemoly-

sis is occurred slowly and then abruptly, discharging hemoglobin into the extracellular medium. The ice channel between the ice crystals fused to form a bigger ice crystal during the thawing process, which was called "recrystallization" by LUYET (1965). The recrystallization described in this book will be called a migratory recrystallization or grain growth which consists in the growth of the large crystals in a group at the expense of small ones as a result of the migration of molecules or atoms (LUYET 1966).

Freezing of red cells suspended in a 39% glycerol solution

Various types of ice crystals were formed in a 39% glycerol solution as shown in Figs. 11, 12, 13, 14, and 15. When the cooling rate was slow by the gradient cooling the ice crystals grew branches from the cool end to the other to form hexagonal structures. When the cooling velocity was increased by use of the circumstance cooling, the coarse spherulites appeared and radiated in all directions from centers of crystallization. An extremely rapid cooling rates by the instantaneous cooling, evanescent spherulites arose. Because the molecules are unable to complete the process of crystallization; they leave the task unfinished in the form of evanescent spherulites (LUYET and RAPATZ 1958, LUYET 1960, cited from MERYMAN 1966).

The red cells treated with glycerol showed a slight and transitory shrinkage without hemolysis as shown in Figs. 12, 13 and 14 during the freeze-thaw process at temperatures ranging from 0°C to 80°C. The cooling rate was about 40°C per minute while the rewarming rate was 10–20°C. It was impossible to detect intracellular ice

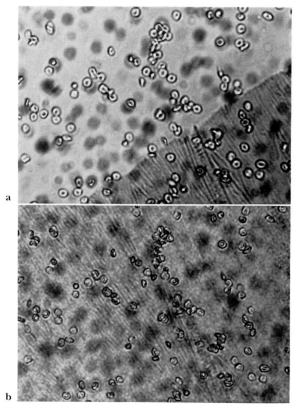

a

b

Fig. 14   Films of red cells suspended in 13% glycerol (HUGGINS' solution) frozen at −35°C to −45°C.
a and **b**: Frozen at a rate of about 30°C to 40°C per minute near the cooling plate. Glass-like fine ice crystals were formed.

crystals by our cryomicroscope. When we observed the freezing process of red cells by 16 mm movie film, we could find the change in color or the change in light transmission. As previously mentioned, this indicated intracellular crystallization or ruptured red cell membrane discharging hemoglobin.

SMITH (1951) observed rabbit blood at −40°C, LUYET (1965) observed human blood at −20°C, and NEI (1967) observed rabbit at −10°C with their original cryomicroscopes; however, there have been no respect of photographs of the freezing process of red cells taken at the temperature of −80°C.

We observed the freeze-thaw process of the red cells suspended in other media with-

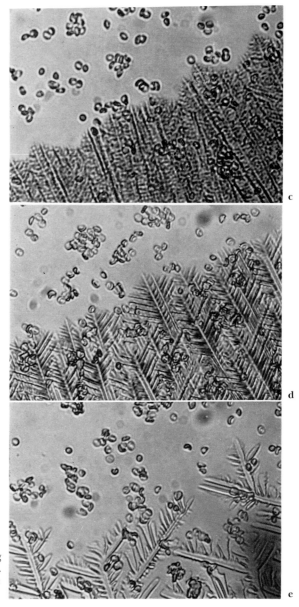

c–e: The more distant from the cooling plate, the larger the ice crystals formed. No hemolysis was seen. *Magnification:* ×400.

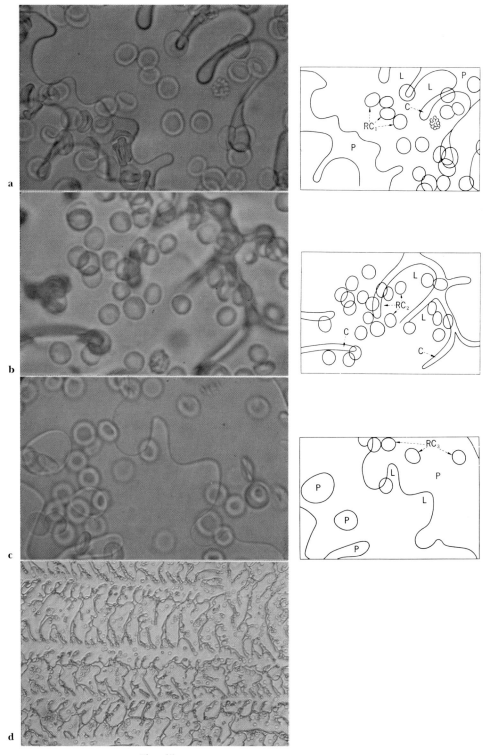

Fig. 15

out glycerol. The ice crystals formed in the 12% hydroxyethyl starch (HES) and in the 6% PVP solution resembled those formed in the glycerol solution when the cooling rate was rapid: however, the ice crystals resembled those formed in the 0.9% saline solution, and the red cells resulted in hemolysis when the cooling rate was 20–40°C per minute. The ice crystals formed in a 39% DMSO solution were very similar to those formed in the glycerol solution, producing neither hemolysis nor morphological changes of the red cells.

LOW POWER ELECTRONMICROSCOPIC OBSERVATION

The red cells to be observed were processed by the procedure reported by my co-worker Ko (1969). Red cells were artificially hemolyzed in water and centrifuged to get sediments consisting of cellular membrane. The same volume of phosphate buffer

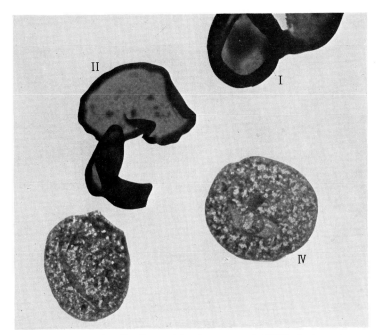

Fig. 16   Frozen red cells observed by low power (×5000) electronmicroscope.

Fig. 15   Changes observed when a film of blood in a final concentration of 40% glycerol according to Huggins, at about −40°C by the gradient cooling and cooled to −80°C, is gradually warmed to about −30°C. As the temperature is slowly raised, the ice blocks decrease in size, and the channels of unfrozen glycerol-plasma widen. **C**, channels of unfrozen plasma-glycerol mixture; **L**, "lobes of ice"; **P**, pools of unfrozen fluid; **RC₂**, red cells shrinked and still smooth-surfaced at −80°C; **RC₃**, red cells reassumed the original shapes at −20°C. *Magnification*: ×800. At lower magnifications, these sheets can be identified as lobes of dendritic structures, as shown in Fig. 11-a, b and Fig. 13.
d: A film of red cells in 40% glycerol (Huggins' solution) frozen at −40°C and cooled to −70°C by the gradient cooling, a meshwork of ice was formed. The cells are buried in or under the ice or condined in channels between the ice. Plasmolysis and deplasmolysis are very slight as well as Figs. 13 and 14. *Magnification*: ×400

(pH = 7.4) was added to the remaining cell debris. Two % OsO$_4$ was also added, and the temperature was kept constant at +4°C. The mixture containing cell debris was dropped on the collodion membrane by pipette and dried for 24 hours before observing with the electronmicroscope (Hitachi B-11 type). At a magnification of × 5000, it was impossible to see the subcellular structures of frozen red cells; however, the following results were obtained from the morphological changes of red cell membrane. Frozen red cells were classified in four types from I to IV according to the aging-like changes of the membrane surface during the freeze-thaw process (Fig. 16). Table 1 shows the classification of fresh, ACD, and frozen red cells, of which ACD red cells had been preserved at 4°C for 2–3 weeks, and frozen red cells had been preserved at −80°C for several weeks by the slow-freeze procedure of HUGGINS.

Type I had much hemoglobin attached to the membrane, while type II had less hemoglobin content at the membrane. Type IV had many holes and/or no hemoglobin at the membrane. Types II and III were intermediate betwen types I and IV. The above-mentioned evidence has been already reported by SUMIDA (1968) and his coworker Ko (1971). We believe that these classifications were caused by the aging of red cells. Young red cells have a greater resistance against low temperature and processing than the old or aged cells.

Table 1   Changes of percent distribution of each group during preservation, observed by low power electronmicroscope.*

Remarks	Classification			
	I	II	III	IV
1. ACD red cells just after collection	50%	20%	20%	10%
2. ACD red cells stored at 4°C for 2–3 weeks	17%	26%	27%	30%
3. HUGGINS' preserved red cells at −80°C for 3 weeks	8%	9%	34%	49%

* Changes from 1 to 2 fit the aging phenomenon, and those from 1 to 3 the aging-like phenomenon. Group I cells decreased either by storage in liquid state at +4°C or by slow-freeze preservation, and in reverse group IV increased.

Hemoglobin attaches too strongly to excoriate the younger cell membrane. Therefore, as shown in Table 1, type I cells occupied 50%, type II 20%, type III 20%, and type IV 10% in fresh ACD red cells. After 2–3 weeks of preservation of these ACD red cells at 4°C, remarkable changes in this percentage were seen: type I decreased to 17%, and type IV increased to 30%, as shown in Table 1. Each intermediate type of red cells also increased as well. We felt that these changes were caused by the aging phenomena of the red blood cells under an aphysiologic situation. Even the red blood cells in 1–2 weeks after collection showed the same changes when they were processed by HUGGINS' procedure.

Type I red cells decreased remarkably while types III and IV increased, which indicated the aging phenomena by the slow-freeze procedures. It might be postulated that these changes were caused by freeze-injury itself and the effect of deglycerolization wash with a large amount of glucose and fructose solution. We called this phenomenon "an aging-like change" of red cells by freeze preservation. Therefore, type

IV cells, which had no hemoglobin at the membrane with small holes from freeze-injury, increased to 40% by frozen blood processing.

Considering the above-mentioned data (Table 1), fresh red cells should be used as early as possible after collection for freeze preservation, because the red cells would become old and fragile during preservation at $4°C$ and easily release hemoglobin. We have experienced several cases of hemoglobinuria from frozen blood transfusion, when we freeze-preserved packed red cells at the second and third week after collection. And, we concluded that red cells should be frozen within the 7th day after collection, if possible immediately after blood-collection.

BIOCHEMISTRY OF FROZEN RED CELLS

Glycerol has no direct toxic action upon red cells. The only effect of glycerol is an osmotic pressure which is caused by the difference of permeability of water and glycerol through the cell membrane. The osmotic pressure produced by those mechanisms acts on both sides of the membrane at various temperatures. Glycerolization and deglycerolization produce no change in the isoagglutinability of red blood cells.

WALLACH et al. (1962), ZEMP et al. (1960), and TULLIS et al. (1966) reported that red cells lost considerable potassium during the freeze-thaw and deglycerolization process, and immediately gained it back intracellularly during the rewarming process at $+37°C$. Potassium concentration of red cells measured by us was 110 mEq per L before processing and 94 mEq per L after the deglycerolization wash (Fig. 43). Thus frozen red cells having a low concentration of intracellular potassium may well have acted as potassium sponges when they are transfused into the patients with hyperkalemia. We prefer the transfusion of washed or frozen red cells to the banked ACD blood for the patient with acute renal failure for the above-mentioned reasons.

As red cells have no intracellular structure except an outer cell membrane, the nature of the red cell membrane and the metabolism of hemoglobin and ATP have frequently been discussed. Energy needed for potassium and sodium exchange is produced by hydrolysis of ATP by ATP-ase. Decrease of ATP has an important factor for maintenance of the membrane function of red cells. The decrease of ATP of red cells occurred at the 8th–10th day after collection when preserved in an ACD medium at $+4°C$. When inosine and/or adenine were added, the decrease of ATP and 2, 3-diphosphoglyceric acid recovered near the normal level, and the life span of red cells was prolonged (NAKAO et al., 1959, YOSHIKAWA et al., 1962). NAKAO and YOSHIKAWA acknowledged that the morphological change from biconcave to spherical shape during preservation was improved by including the above-mentioned additives. ATP content of red cell is a good parameter to indicate the physiological and morphological integrity of the red cells. There are many research workers currently discussing frozen red cells from these metabolic points of view.

SLOW-FREEZE PRESERVATION OF RED CELLS
(Standard method of frozen blood transfusion in Japan)

Packed red cells

Blood was collected as ACD blood from the donors, and erythrocytes were usually separated on the 5th day after collection of the blood. The packed red cells were pro-

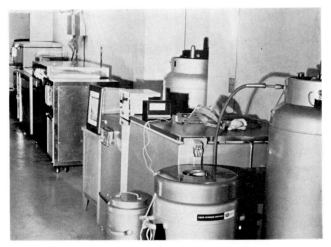

Fig. 17   Frozen blood section, Medical low temperature unit, the National Fukuoka Central Hospital, 1972.

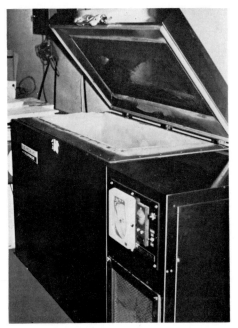

Fig. 18   Deep freezer (−80°C) convenient for high humidity climate in Japan.

cessed as frozen blood within 12 hours. However, as more fresh erythrocytes are frozen, higher recovery rates are produced, as will be seen later.

Cryoprotective agent

A 79.2% glycerol solution was used according to the procedure of HUGGINS, C. E. (1966). Constitution of HUGGINS' solution was as follows:

Glycerol	79.2%
Glucose	8.2%
Fructose	1.0%
EDTA	0.3%

Deep freezer

The total capacity of the deep freezers at the National Fukuoka Central Hospital

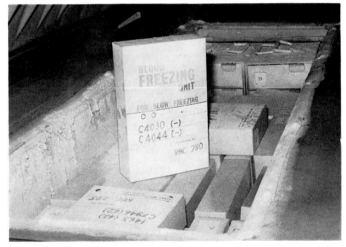

Fig. 19   Blood freezing unit in a deep freezer at −80°C, the National Fukuoka
Central Hospital, 1972.

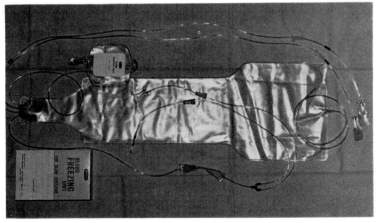

Fig. 20   SUMIDA's blood freezing unit for slow freezing.

is 1000 units of blood.   There are five freezers, each with a capacity of 250 to 350 liters
(Figs. 17, 18, and 19).

Blood freezing container

Sumida's blood freezing container for slow freezing was used in this series of frozen
blood transfusions.   The container is constructed as shown in Figs. 20, 21, and 22, and

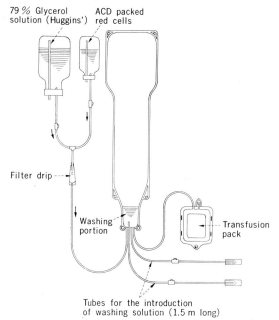

Fig. 21   Sumida's blood freezing unit for the slow-freeze procedure
by use of Huggins' 79% glycerol solution.

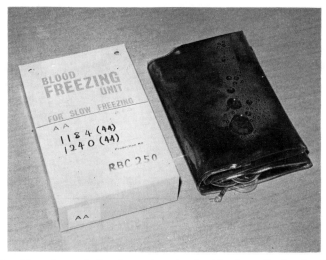

Fig. 22   Sumida's freezing unit, primed with glycerolized red cells.

is made of polyvinylchloride film which is durable for the freeze preservation of red cells at −110°C. Freeze-processing of red cells as well as washing without freezing them is performed *best* in a closed system by use of this container sterilized with ethylene oxide. The container is constructed with two bags. One is a main container for freeze preservation of glycerolized red cells, and the other is a smaller bag used for

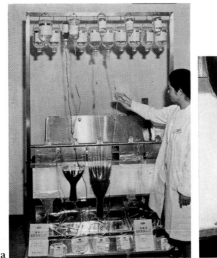
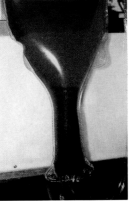

a   b

Fig. 23   SUMIDA's cytoglomerator.

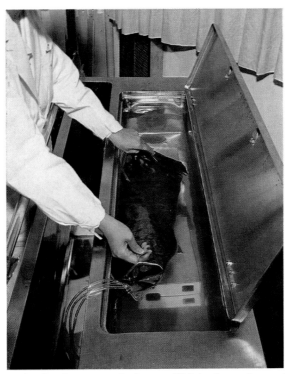

Fig. 24   Thawing in a water bath at +40°C by SUMIDA's cytoglomerator.

transferring thawed deglycerolized red cells. The bags are connected with a plastic tube. The main container has two portions, as shown in Fig. 21. The dilated portion is for decanting the washing solution, and the narrow portion is for glycerolizing and washing the red cells. Four tubes are attached at the entrance of the washing portion, and they are plugged in by small balls. Each small ball is released and pushed into the washing portion before use. A filter drip which can be used for glycerolization is attached to one of the tubes and is divided into Y-shaped tubes, and red cells and glycerol solution are introduced into the container through the filter drip. A blood transfer bag is attached to one of the other three tubes. The two remaining tubes are used for deglycerolization wash, and one of them protrudes 5 cm inside beyond the entrance of the main container.

Apparatus for deglycerolization and refrigerated centrifuge

(1) SUMIDA's cytoglomerator consists of a 40–45°C water bath and a hanger to hold the container (Figs. 23, and 24). This cytoglomerator is a modification of HUGGINS' original apparatus (Fig. 25).

(2) A refrigerated centrifuge (Sorvall RC3) with swinging four buckets of 1000 g capacity at 3000 rpm (about 3500 gravity or more) was used in our experiments.

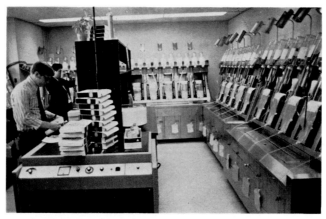

Fig. 25   HUGGINS' cytoglomerator at surgical low temperature unit, MGH., Boston.

Procedures

Measurement of packed red cells : Weight of packed red cells was measured and expressed in milliliters (m*l*). A small sample of the packed red cells (0.02 m*l*) was taken to measure hemoglobin concentration.

Glycerolization : A blood freezing container was placed on the hanger of the cytoglomerator (Fig. 23). The red blood cells were introduced through a spike needle on the tip of the Y-shaped tube, followed by the addition of a 79.2% glycerol solution through the other needle. Mixing of the glycerol solution and red blood cells could be assisted manually by compression and release on the main bag. It took about 15 minutes to complete the glycerolization, after which the tube was ligated. The container with glycerolized red cells was folded up and packed into a cardboard box (Fig. 22), which was frozen in a deep freezer at $-80°C$ to $-110°C$ (Fig. 19).

Thawing and deglycerolization : The container of frozen blood was thawed in 2–3 minutes in a water bath at 40–45°C (Fig. 24). Thawed glycerolized red cells were collected to the washing portion of the container and the container was then placed on the hanger.

An equal volume of a 50% glucose solution was introduced gradually to the thawed glycerolized red cells in the container through a tube. Subsequently, 2000 ml of 5% fructose solution were added through two tubes. Red cells in the concentrated non-ionic solution were aggregated and precipitated around the washing portion of the container. The agglomerated red cells were disaggregated and washed by a 5% fructose solution flowing into the container from a height of 1.5 meter H_2O. This phenomenon of agglomeration was explained by C. E. HUGGINS (1963) as shown in Fig. 26.

The most important and interesting part of HUGGINS' report is the method of deglycerolization by use of red cell agglomeration. The reversible agglomeration phenomenon occurs in a non-electrolyte solution of pH between 5.2 and 6.1, and the agglomerated red cell masses are precipitated in the narrowed inlet portion of the main bag, but they are easily resuspended by an elevation of pH or by the addition of an electrolyte solution (Fig. 26).

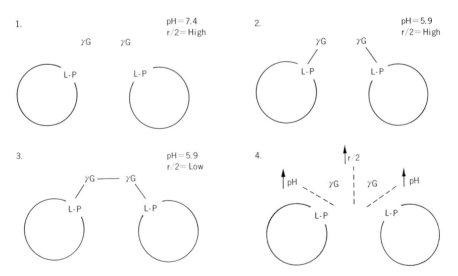

Fig. 26 Reversible agglomeration of erythrocytes, and resuspension of agglomerated cells (HUGGINS, C. E., 1963).

As one of the tubes protruded 5 cm beyond the container, it was convenient to wash the red cells floating at the upper portion of the container. After the introduction of 2000 ml of 5% fructose solution, agglomerated red cells were completely settled in several minutes. Usually this took about 5 minutes. The supernatant solution containing hemolyzed cell debris, free hemoglobin and glycerol was decanted into the dilated portion of the container located at the other side of the hanger by shifting the folded portion of the container. This is shown in Fig. 27, which describes the entire slow-

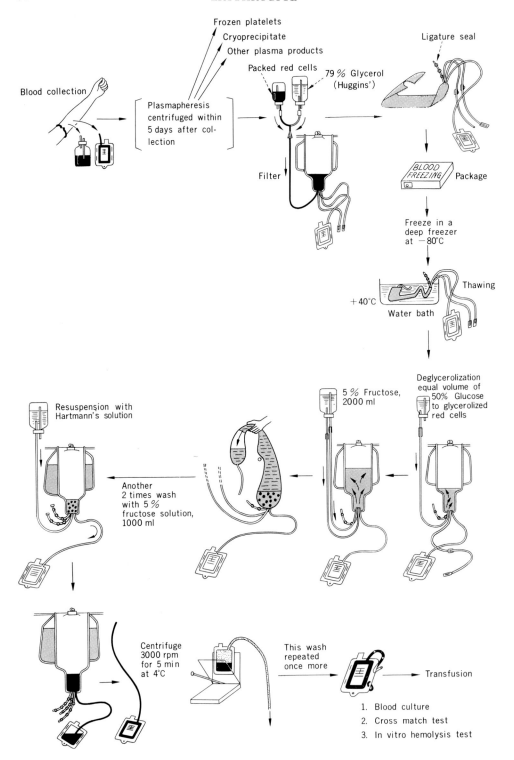

Fig. 27   Slow-freeze procedure using Sumida's blood freezing unit, modified from Huggins, C. E.

freeze procedure as it is conducted at the National Fukuoka Central Hospital. The second wash was done with 1000 ml of 5% fructose solution. Each supernatant was decanted as perfectly as possible. Precipitated red cells were transferred into the blood transfer bag, and about 200 ml of 0.9% saline solution were added in order to resuspend the agglomerated red cells. Resuspended frozen red cells in a blood transfer bag were centrifuged by 2000 rpm (1120 G) for 10 minutes to separate and decant the supernatant containing free hemoglobin and remaining glycerol. In order to wash out those solutes as much as possible, the final wash with 200 ml of 0.9% saline was repeated once more and the supernatant was also decanted. When the frozen red cells washed two extra times with 0.9% saline were transfused into the patients, post-transfusion increment of free hemoglobin in the recipient serum was very slight and a large amount of frozen red cells for transfusion could be available (Fig. 28).

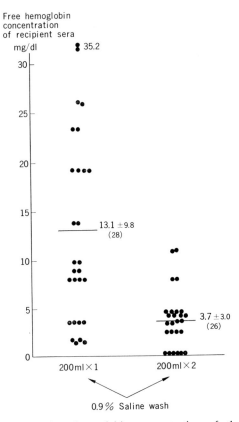

Fig. 28 Plasma free hemoglobin concentration of the recipient increased very slight after one unit of frozen red cells washed by two times with 200 ml of 0.9% saline.

Pre-transfusion examination of frozen red cells: A small sample of processed resuspended red cells was left at 38°C for 30 minutes, and the supernatant free hemoglobin concentration was examined before and after incubation. When the supernatant hemoglobin concentration of the frozen red cells increases over 1500 mg per dl after

ABO BLOOD GROUP	CODE GOT
Rh TYPE	DONOR

COLLECTED: 19 _____ ,   THAWED: 19 _____

FROZEN: 19 _____

    PACKED CELLS: _____ ml(gm) Hb _____ g/dl

    8.6 M GLYCEROL SOLUTION: Wt. _____ , LOT # _____

    28% GLYCEROL SOLUTION: Wt. _____ , LOT # _____

DEGLYCEROLIZATION: 50% GLUCOSE _____ , 5% FRUCTOSE _____

                      20% MANNITOL+0.9% SALINE _____ + _____

                      0.9% SALINE _____ ml×_____

PROCESSED CELLS _____ gm(ml) Hb _____ g/dl

SUPERNATANT CHEMISTRIES	ELECTROLYTES (mEq/L)	CULTURE
FREE HEMOGLOBIN (mg/dl) RESUSPENDED _____ 1. _____ 2. _____ INCUBATED _____ 3. _____ 4. _____	K _____ Ca _____ Na _____ Mg _____ Cl _____	examined after 9 days and "no growth"

O	A	B	AB	D	C	E	c	e	K	k	F_y^a	F_y^b	P	JK^a	JK^b	M	N	S	s	L_e^a	L_e^b	L_u^a	L_u^b

RECIPIENT	ABO BLOOD GROUP
SEX AGE	Rh TYPE

DIAGNOSIS

TRANSFUSION	REACTION (BAD EFFECT)

UNIT(S)

PREVIOUS TRANSFUSION: BANKED ACD BLOOD

                             FROZEN FLOOD

REMARK(S):   SHORTAGE, EMERGENCY, TRANSFUSION REACTION, ORGAN TRANSPLANTATION, RENAL INSUFFICIENCY, RARE TYPE, OTHERS _____ ,

NATIONAL FUKUOKA CENTRAL HOSPITAL, FROZEN BLOOD SECTION

Fig. 29   Frozen blood transfusion records.
Upper: the first half. *Lower*: the reverse.

incubation, those frozen red cells should not be used, because the osmotic fragility of the red cells might also be increased. Another small sample of frozen red cells was taken to test the bacterial culture and examined to show no "growth" after 9 days. All of these examined data were recorded on the card (Fig. 29).

Metabolic additives: Adenosinetriphosphate (Adetphos®), α-tocopherol acetate (Juvera®, Vitamin E), Hypoxanthine riboside (Inosine, Inosie®), and Glutathione (Glutide®) as supplements to cryoprotectants. Attempts have already been made to improve the viability and survival of stored blood by addition of metabolic additives

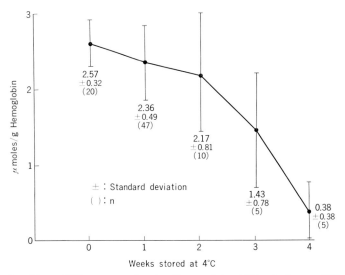

Fig. 30 ATP content of red cells stored in ACD solution at 4°C.

such as inosine, guanosine, and adenine to the anticoagulant ACD solution. Such purine nucleosides had been used for the preservation of blood in the liquid state.

GABRIO et al. (1955) first reported that the decreased content of ATP and 2,3-diphosphoglyceric acid during storage was restored to some extent by incubation with inosine and adenosine, and that the ability of these cells to survive in the circulation after transfusion was also improved. They also determined that inosine was well metabolized by human erythrocytes and supported active cation influx. GABRIO et al. (1956) constituted Acid-Citrate-Dextrose-Inosine (ACDI) solution as a preservative medium for blood during storage in the liquid state at 4°C. However, NAKAO et al. (1959) reported that the ATP level of human red cells was not increased any longer by addition of inosine alone after storage at 4°C for 8 weeks. They confirmed that neither adenine, adenosine, AMP, nor ADP was effective when added separately, and that combined use of adenine and inosine only increased the ATP level of the red cells. They suggested that ATP in the erythrocytes played a role in maintaining the disk shape of the red cells.

Considering their comprehensive studies on the storage of blood, a new preservative ACD medium containing inosine 10 g per liter and adenine sulfate 2.5 g per liter was introduced to maintain the ATP level and the osmotic resistance of red cells (NAKAO

et al., 1960).   Erythrocytes preserved in "ACDIA" medium showed a high viability for
a long time after transfusion (WADA et al., 1960).   STRUMIA (1965) investigated the loss
of adenosinetriphosphate (ATP) in erythrocytes subjected to freezing and thawing.
This was also measured by us, and is shown in Figs. 31 and 32.   Loss of ATP has been
one of the most constant manifestations of damage to red cells in ACD blood stored at
4°C, as shown in Fig. 30.   STRUMIA (1966) found that there was little difference in the
effect of adenine and inosine whether added before or after freezing and thawing.
Inosine alone improved recovery of ATP, but only in the presence of buffered electrolytes.   Adenine alone had no effect on ATP recovery, but there was regeneration of
ATP upon incubation with adenine in the presence of buffered electrolytes.   VALERI
et al. (1967) applied adenine (0.6 mM per liter) supplementation of glycerolized red
cells prior to freezing, which caused insignificant change in the *in vivo* or *in vitro*

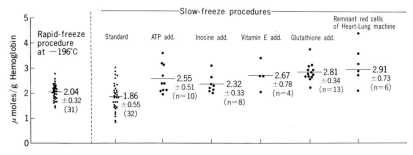

Fig. 31   ATP content of frozen red cells.

Table   2   Effects of supplemental additives on recovery rates and
ATP contents of freeze-preserved red cells.

Remarks		Recovery rate (%)	ATP content (micro moles/g Hb)
Slow-freeze procedure (HUGGINS)		**72.8**±10.4 (n=50)	**1.86**±0.55 (n=32)
Rapid-freeze procedure (ROWE)		**82.9**±12.5 (n=50)	**2.04**±0.32 (n=31)
Slow-freeze procedure (HUGGINS) +	ATP	**75.9**±16.6 (n=30)	**2.55**±0.51 (n=10)
	Inosine	**83.6**± 9.6 (n=34)	**2.32**±0.33 (n= 8)
	Vitamin E	**77.8**±13.0 (n=38)	**2.67**±0.78 (n= 4)
	Glutathione	**75.6**±18.9 (n=19)	**2.81**±0.34 (n=13)
Slow-freeze procedue (HUGGINS) by use of remnant blood in heart-lung machine after cardiac surgery		**80.6**±14.8 (n= 4)	**2.91**±0.73 (n= 6)

±:   Standard deviation.

characteristics of erythrocytes stored at temperatures ranging from 4°C to −20°C.   One
of these metabolic additives was added to one unit of the packed red cells before glycerolization in this series of clinical surveys, and the effectiveness of the supplemental
additives was measured from the recovery rate and ATP content of red cells.   The
doses were 80 mg of ATP, 200 mg of Vitamin E, 400 mg of Inosine or 200 mg of Glutathione for each unit.   The recovery rate of each series was compared with that of red

cells processed by the standard slow-freeze procedure. ATP content of processed red cells with the prefreeze-addition of ATP was measured and compared with that of red cells by the standard slow-freeze procedure (Figs. 30, 31, 32, and Table 2). ATP content of red cells just after collection as ACD blood was 2.57 μmoles per gram Hemoglobin, that in the 5th day to 7th day after collection was 2.36 μmoles per gram Hemoglobin; that of the rapid-freeze red cells after ROWE's procedure without ATP addition was 2.04 μmoles per gram Hemoglobin, and that of the slow-freeze red cells added ATP was 2.55 μmoles per gram Hemoglobin. On the other hand, ATP content of red cells in the 4th week after collection was 0.38 μmoles per gram Hemoglobin, showing a remarkable decrease of ATP in the ACD red cells preserved at 4°C. The recovery rates of those processed red cells are shown in Table 2. The recovery rate of the controls was 72.8 ± 10.4 (n =50)%, that of the Inosine series was 83.6 ± 9.6 (n = 24)% and that of the Glutathione series was 75.6 ± 18.9 (n = 19)%.

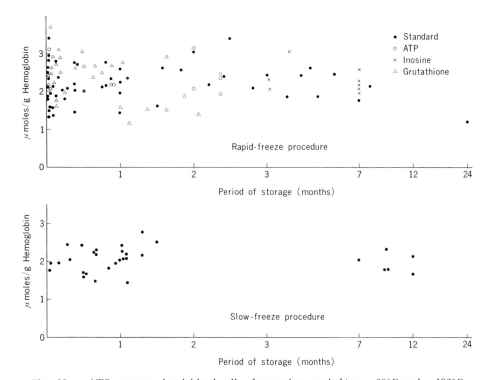

Fig. 32   ATP content of red blood cells after various periods at $-80°C$ and $-196°C$.

KUROKAWA et al. (1968, 1969) reported that Vitamin E was also effective in prolonging the preservation period of ACD blood in a liquid state. In this study the author used Inosine, Vitamin E, ATP, and Glutathion instead of adenine to increase the recovery rate of HUGGINS' preserved red cells, examining those agents from the following points of view: (a) cryoprotective effects of those agents, (b) effectiveness in preserving ATP content of red cells, and (c) effectiveness in preserving the integrity of red cell membranes.

The freezing process of red cells suspended in 0.9% saline solution containing ATP was observed by a cryomicroscope (Nikon NE type, previously mentioned). However, no direct action for cryoprotection was observed. In the slow-freeze procedure, the ATP content of frozen red cells decreased less in those red cells in the ATP series than in those processed by the standard slow-freeze procedure. This finding indicated that red cells could be preserved more effectively in the frozen state when ATP was added before glycerolization. This was confirmed by the increase in recovery rate from 73% to 76% when ATP was added in the packed red cells before glycerolization. Also the recovery rate further increased up to 83.6% by use of Inosine. These data showed that red cells could be preserved better in the frozen state by the additional use of ATP, Vitamin E, Inosine or Glutathione. However, there were no positive data to indicate whether or not these agents had direct cryoprotective action. The author believes that these agents actively prevented the decrease of intracellular ATP and exerted an indirect action to preserve the functional integrity of the red cell membrane not in the frozen state but in the liquid state.

IWAN W. D. HENDERSON (1970) also reported that ATP would be effective in preserving red cells in the frozen state from his basic research. However, he did not report his findings from the clinical point of view. Vitamin E increased the recovery rate of red cells, and the author agreed with a report by KÖRNER et al. (1965) that Vitamin E lessened the increase of osmotic fragility of erythrocytes and played a role in maintaining the normal biconcave shape to preserve the structural-chemical integrity of the red cell membrane.

A simple washing of red cells

Packed red cells can be washed with 5% fructose solution without freeze preservation. The ACD red cells should be used within 10 days after collection for this purpose. Resuspension is done with 0.9% saline solution. Fifty % glucose solution should not be used for the first wash if the red cells are not frozen with addition of 79% glyc-

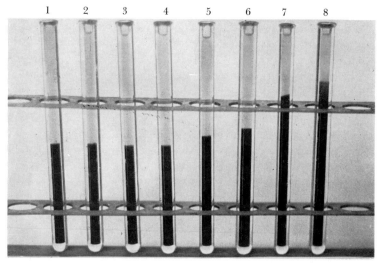

Fig. 33   Same volume of packed red cells was added to each solution (1 and 2: 0.9% saline, 3 and 4: 5% xylitol in water, 5 and 6: 5% fructose in water, and 7 and 8: 5% glucose in water), and then left for 60 minutes at room temperature.

erol solution. The packed ACD red cells are introduced into the SUMIDA's container, and the first wash is started with 5% fructose solution. After three washes with 5% fructose solution, red cells are resuspended with 0.9% saline solution and transfused immediately. Wash with 5% *glucose* solution should be prohibited as it causes remarkable swelling of red cells (Fig. 33) and those red cells will be intravascularly hemolyzed and produce massive hemoglobinuria after transfusion.

Slow-freeze preservation with DMSO

In general, the cryoprotective compounds should have the following properties: (a) low molecular weight, (b) good solubility in salt solution, (c) transparent to red cell membrane (LOVELOCK, 1959). The molecular weight of DMSO is 78, it is completely soluble in a salt-water systems, and it rapidly penetrates the cell membranes. DMSO was introduced early as cryoprotective agent of red cells by LOVELOCK and BISHOP (1959). HUGGINS (1963) used 8.6 M DMSO in 8–10% sucrose solution as a cryoprotective medium for the slow-freeze preservation of a large volume of red cells. About 600 ml of packed red cells were mixed with the DMSO solution in a polyvinylchloride container of 1000 ml capacity, which was frozen in a deep freezer at −85°C or in a dry ice box at −75°C. Thawing was accomplished in a water bath at +40°C. The recovery rate of red cells was 82%, and the concentration of DMSO decreased to 1.5% after

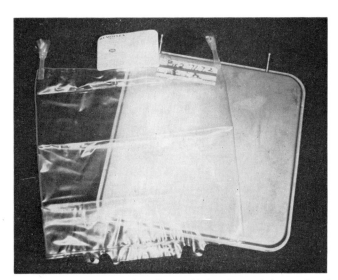

Fig. 34   Blood freezing container for rapid freezing, stainless steel and plastic sheet.

washout. DMSO is relatively non-toxic, and 13 g per kg body weight of DMSO can be intravenously infused to canines without any harm. HUGGINS (1964, 1965) used 133 units of the frozen red cells processed by the method previously mentioned for 39 patients. He preserved red cells in the frozen state by use of glycerol and propylene glycol, of which 360 units were transfused into 65 patients: however, he is now using only glycerol as a cryoprotectant. Ethylene glycol was also tested, and there was no clinical use for it.

Other cryoprotective substance for red cells

In the early days, 10–30% glycerol was used for the cryoprotection of red cells (WOODCOCK et al., 1941, FLORIO, 1943). The relatively rapid-freezing procedure for preservation of red cells was also performed. However, it was not possible to preserve a large enough volume of blood in the frozen state for transfusion by this method. VINOGRAD-FINKEL (1958) reported a study on the freeze preservation of red blood cells in the Soviet Union by use of ethanol and another carbohydrate as cryoprotectants. BLACKSHAW (1954) used glycol sugar and amide as cryoprotectants for red cells, at various speeds of freezing. BRICKA and BESSIS (1955) used several substances with high molecular weights, and SLOVITER (1962) tried 30% polyoxyethylene solution for the preservation of red cells. Their recovery rate was 83%, which was unexpectedly good, and the *in vivo* survival was 85% at 24 hours after transfusion. MERYMAN (1966) noticed that the recovery rate would gradually decrease during preservation at −79°C. Fifty or more cryoprotectants are shown in a comprehensive review by KAROW (1969).

RAPID-FREEZE PRESERVATION OF RED CELLS

The author used the rapid-freeze procedure (ROWE, 1968) for the preservation of red cells in the frozen state according to A. W. ROWE's procedure (1968), which was modified from KRIJNEN (1965). Seven days after collection as ACD blood, the same volume of 28% v/v glycerol solution was added to the packed red cells in a plastic bag of 600 ml capacity, and they were well mixed to a final glycerol concentration of 14%. Glyce-

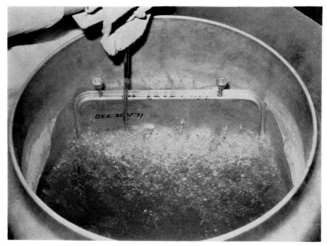

Fig. 35   Glycerolized red cells in a stainless steel container is frozen in liquid
nitrogen.

rolized red cells were introduced into a stainless or a plastic container (Fig. 35) holding approximately 600 ml, which was frozen in liquid nitrogen.

The outer sleeve-cap was removed from the neck tube of the stainless steel container and replaced with a new one, and the rubber stoppers were held in place by metal capseals. The blood-glycerol mixture was frozen by immersion of the container in an upright position into a pool of liquid nitrogen (Fig. 36). The liquid nitrogen boiled vigorously for 2 to 3 minutes and subsided when the freezing process of the glycerolized red cells was accomplished. The containers were stored in an upright position in a liquid nitrogen refrigerator. The rubber capped neck tubes should not be stored under the liquid phase of liquid nitrogen but they should project above the liquid into the gaseous phase. The preservation temperature should be held at $-150°C$ (liquid nitrogen gas phase) to $-196°C$ (liquid nitrogen) (Fig. 37), and should not be preserved in any mechanical deep freezer of $-80°C$ to $-97°C$, because the ice crystals formed in 14% glycerol solution will physically change at the temperature of a mechan-

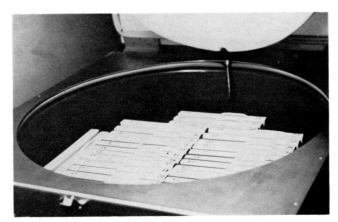

Fig. 36   Liquid nitrogen stocker for storage of rapid-freeze red cells.

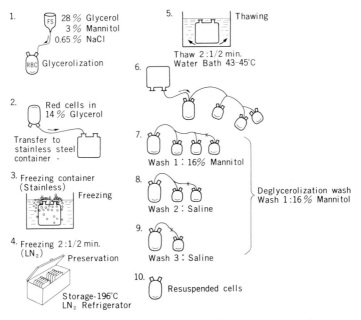

Fig. 37   Rapid-freeze preservation of red cells (ROWE, A. W., 1969).

ical freezer and recrystallize to provoke hemolysis. Thawing was accomplished by immersing the entire container with agitation for 2–3 minutes in a 45°C water bath.

The thawed blood was transferred by gravity from the metal container into a plastic bag, and then centrifuged at 3000 rpm (2510 G) at 4°C for 5 minutes for deglycerolization wash. After centrifugation, the supernatant containing free hemoglobin and glycerol were removed before introduction of the first washing solution. The first wash was done by 400 ml of 16% manntol in a 0.9% saline solution. The bag was thoroughly mixed and centrifuged at 3000 rpm for 5 minutes. The supernatant was again removed and the free hemoglobin concentration was measured. This was followed by two 400 ml of the 0.9% saline solution to remove cell debris and free hemoglobin. Free hemoglobin concentration of these two supernatants were also measured. The frozen red cells were transfused as packed cells resuspended in 0.9% saline or in hemologous or autologous plasma. The total rapid-freeze procedure is shown in Fig. 35 (ROWE, 1968).

PRE- AND POST-TRANSFUSION EXAMINATION

Preservation of human red cells is considered to be satisfactory when the red cells are circulating and functioning immediately after transfusion. Therefore, it will be important to test the freeze-preserved red cells before and after transfusion.

This chapter deals with the methods of examination by the author to determine whether or not the freeze-preserved red cells can be used for transfusion. In 1965, when HUGGINS, C. E. introduced "Frozen Blood Transfusion" to Japan, he also published several noteworthy papers on the same subject. However, there was no description of the viability criterion of the processed red cells before transfusion. The author would like to present several criteria of frozen red cells in this chapter.

Macroscopic differentiation of frozen red cells

Slow-freeze-preserved red cells : If the container has a microhole, water in the thawing bath will be stained with blood. Both the blood and the container must be discarded. Usually freeze-thawed red cells precipitate as an agglomerated mass (reversible agglomeration) during the introduction of 2000 ml of 5% fructose solution. However, in some cases it has happened that no agglomeration could be seen even 10 minutes or more after the 5% fructose solution had been totally introduced. It is assumed that those red cells had been processed improperly, probably at the glycerolization stage and they should also be discarded. However, the additional use of another 500 ml of 5% fructose solution might be recommended, as such phenomena were seen when the volume of 5% fructose solution was too short to provoke agglomeration. Therefore, the volume of packed red cells should be recorded on the cardboard box, as this facilities exact calculation of the volume of 50% glucose and 5% fructose solution which should be used for the deglycerolization wash.

Rapid-freeze-preserved red cells : If there was a leakage due to improper sealing of the inlet part of the stainless steel container, the liquid nitrogen which leaked into it evaporated during thawing and dilated the container like a balloon to blow off the seal. Red cells in those containers would have been hemolyzed and contaminated, and therefore could not be used for transfusion, so they would be discarded.

Measurements of hemoglobin

High concentration :   Hemoglobin concentration of packed red cells was measured both before and after processing.   Since the concentration was very high, it should be well mixed before measurement.   The sample was taken directly from the blood transfer bottle or pack.   Part of the blood sample (0.02 m*l*) was taken by a micropipette, which was added to 5 m*l* of the reagent (Van Kampenzijlstra's Reagent modified by Matsubara, 1970). After the sample was allowed to stand for usually 30 minutes to one hour at room temperature, the optical densities were determined with the Coleman Jr. II Spectrophotometer, using the cuvettes of 1.0 cm, at the maximum wavelength (541 mμ) and the minimum wavelength (503 mμ) of HgCN.   The optical density (Es) was read and recorded using distilled water as a reference (Estd).

$$\text{Hemoglobin concentration} = \frac{\text{Es}}{\text{Estd}} \times 16 \ (\text{g Hb per } 100 \text{ m} l)$$

Hemoglobin concentration of packed red cells before freezing was 21.0 ± 3.10 (n = 101) g per d*l*, and that of slow-freeze-processed red cells was 27.5 ± 3.7 (n = 36) g per d*l*.   These data show that the processed red cells were remarkably concentrated.

Low concentration of hemoglobin :   Free hemoglobin concentration of plasma, supernatants of decanted washing solution and resuspended red cells were measured as follows.   It was especially difficult to measure the free hemoglobin concentration in plasma when it was 50 mg per d*l* or less, and also difficult when jaundice was present. In those plasma the reproducibility of the data was not satisfactory, and the coefficient of variation (CV) of the measured data was very large, usually 20% or more.   However, as the samples in this series for the measurement of hemoglobin were mostly supernatants of decanted washing solution, the above-mentioned method of Matsubara was applied to get the satisfactory reproducibility.   The benzidin method, which is used in the United States, is preferable to the HgCN method.   The supernatant was centrifuged again at 3000 rpm, 1.0 m*l* of which was added to 5.0 m*l* of the reagent, mixed and allowed to stand for 30 to 60 minutes.   Then the optical density was recorded under the same conditions described above.   Hemoglobin concentration of the resuspended supernatant was 968 ± 357 (n = 24) mg per d*l*, and that of the second wash with 0.9% saline was 275 ± 135 (n = 22) mg per d*l* in the slow-freeze procedure.

The supernatant of rapid-freeze-preserved red cells was again centrifuged, 2.0 m*l* of which were added to the same volume of the reagent, and the optical density was read and recorded at 541 mμ, using the reagent as reference.   The supernatant hemoglobin concentration of the first wash was 239.7 ± 71.0 (n = 6), that of the second wash with 16% mannitol in 0.9% saline was 57.3 ± 23.5 (n = 6), that of the third wash with 0.9% saline was 141.5 ± 44.4 (n = 6), and that of the 4th wash with 0.9% saline was 61.0 ± 30 (n = 6).   Therefore, the supernatant hemoglobin concentration of resuspended red cells just before transfusion was higher in the slow-freeze procedure than in the rapid-freeze procedure.   However, the free hemoglobin actually infused into the patients would be about 100 mg per unit in the slow-freeze procedure and about 40 mg per unit in the rapid-freeze procedure.   These amounts were very small and considered unharmful as the supernatant containing free hemoglobin was centrifuged and mostly discarded before transfusion.   We examined the increases of serum free hemoglobin concentration just after the frozen blood transfusion was process as described above. We observed a very slight increase of serum hemoglobin in several cases as shown in Fig. 38, but there was no case of hemoglobinuria. Some hematologists were anxious about the frozen red cells suspended in a medium with a high concentration of free hemoglobin, because they felt that it was caused from the increased osmotic fragility of frozen red cells. However, such anxiety was unnecessary because it was explained by the hypothesis of the aging-like phenomenon during the freeze-thaw deglycerolization process, which was previously mentioned in the chapter (2) on the low power electronmicroscopic observation of frozen red cells. The *in vivo* life span, osmotic fragility, and ATP content also confirmed the integrity of the processed red cells. They were also more able to tolerate osmotic stress than the ACD red cells in the third week after collection.

In vitro test of hemolysis

A small sample of the resuspended processed red cells in a test tube was incubated in a water bath at 37°C for 30 minutes before transfusion. The free hemoglobin concentration in the supernatant should not increase above 1500 mg per dl. It appears to be one of the most reliable evaluations to prove the safety of the frozen red cells before transfusion. Three thousand units of frozen red cells tested in this way were transfused into 400 or more patients without any harmful side effects.

Leukocyte counts of processed frozen red cells

The leukocyte count of red cells frozen by the slow-freeze procedure was 666 ± 382 (n = 53) per mm^3, and that of those frozen by the rapid-freeze procedure was 183 ± 88 (n = 15) per mm^3. Therefore, the slow-freeze packed cells processed by HUGGINS' procedure contained more in leukocyte counts than those processed by the rapid-freeze

Table 3   The contrast between the biochemical status of resuspended frozen red cells and that of ACD blood stored for 10–20 days at 4°C.

	SUMIDA, 1969			HUGGINS, 1968[2]	
	Slow-freeze	Rapid-freeze	ACD[1]	Frozen slow-freeze	ACD
Na mEq/l	74.4 ± 11.4 (86)	152.8± 0.9 (12)	144	84.3 ±11.6 (50)	154
K mEq/l	3.1 ± 1.1 (86)	0.7± 0.2 (12)	13	1.9 ± 0.62 (50)	23
Cl mEq/l	77.1 ± 8.7 (86)	151.2± 1.2 (12)	69	85.2 ± 9.3 (50)	—
Ca mEq/l	0.98± 0.27 (62)	0.6± 0.1 (12)	1.6	1.4*	8.2*
Mg mEq/l	0.2 ± 0.02 (5)	—	0.7	—	—
Phosphate	—	—	—	1.1*	7.2*
Citrate	—	—	—	0	—
Glucose	—	—	—	4.5 ± 0.6 (g%)	0.3 (g%)
Glycerol	—	—	—	0.22± 0.1 (mM/l)	—
Total protein	≑0	≑0	6.6	≑0	6.0
WBC counts/mm^3	666 ±383 (53)	183 ±89 (15)	3200	650	10150
pH	6.96± 0.13 (5)	—	6.23	7.00	6.0
Anti-A titer	—	—	—	nil to 1 : 8	variable
Anti-B titer	—	—	—	nil to 1 : 8	variable

1) SUMIDA, S.: *Clin. Surge.*, 23: 443, 1968. In Japanese.   *: mg %.
2) HUGGINS, C. E.: Human transplantation, p. 669, 1968.   ( ): n.

procedure of ROWE (Table 3, and Fig. 38). The real reason for this evidence was not resolved. HUGGINS (1964) reported that the leukocyte count of blood frozen by his method was 650 per mm³ after deglycerolization wash using 6 liters of 9% sugar solution; however, he is now washing the thawed red cells with 2 liters of 5% fructose solution, and therefore more leukocytes might remain. Our impression was that the leukocyte counts decreased when the wash with 0.9% saline was repeated.

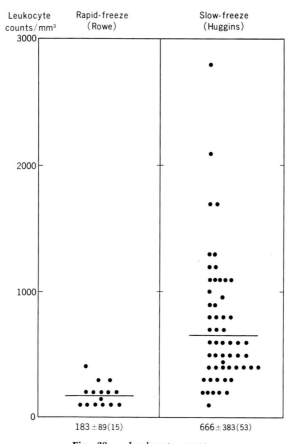

Fig. 38 Leukocyte counts.

Cross match test

As the frozen red cells contain few plasma components, the cross match test was usually satisfied with the major test only. Evidence of mis-matching of the test was not encountered.

In vivo **survival of processed red cells**

Ashby's method : Frozen red cells of group O blood were transfused into patients of A or B group. Red cells of the recipient were precipitated by use of anti-A or -B serum at definite intervals. Following this, the survived was measured by counting unprecipitated red cells. The processed red cells were shown to survive for 90 days to 110 days (Fig. 39).

^{51}Cr method :   The processed red cells were labeled with ^{51}Cr before transfusion. One hundred to 150 μC of $Na_2{}^{51}CrO_4$ were added to a unit of frozen red cells. Red cells were then allowed to stand for an hour at room temperature, and 200 ml of 0.9% saline were added and centrifuged at 2000 rpm.   The supernatant was discarded and the packed frozen red cells were transfused.   In 60 minutes, 4 ml of the first blood sample were collected as reference, and 24 hours later 4.0 ml of the second sample of blood were taken in order to calculate the survival rate at the 24th hour, as several investigators have demonstrated that nonviable red cells that are damaged during preservation are usually removed within the first 24 hours after transfusion (SZYMANSKI et al., 1968, JONES et al., 1957).

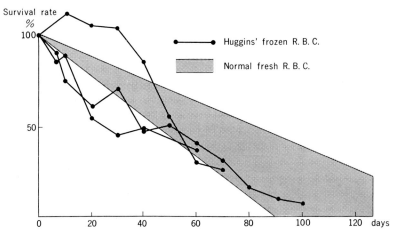

Fig. 39   *In vivo* survival (ASHBY's method) of frozen red cells (F.R.C.) at 24 hours after transfusion.

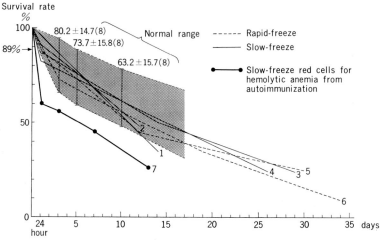

Fig. 40   *In vivo* survival of frozen red cells (F.R.C.) at 24 hours after transfusion (^{51}Cr technique)

Blood samples were collected every week thereafter, and the survival rates of ^{51}Cr red cells were calculated (Fig. 40). The results, given in Fig. 40, show that 89% of the red cells preserved either at −80°C or at −196°C remained in circulation for 24 hours after transfusion. The life span measured by the ^{51}Cr method was shorter than that by ASHBY's method. Volunteers were not used in this series of sudies. The post-transfusion red cell life span was related neither to the freeze-preservation procedures nor to the length of storage in the frozen state within 3 years. These data suggest that the preserved red cells by the slow-freeze and the rapid-freeze procedures at our hospital maintain normal life span. We have to emphasize, in addition, the interrelation between the donor red cells and the recipient's circulating environment since the recipient must be able to restore reversibly damaged red cells.

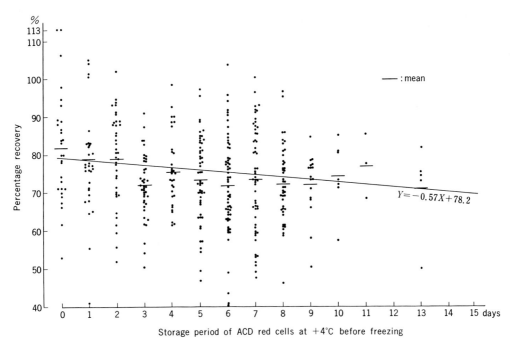

Fig. 41   The regression line shows a negative correlation between the freshness of ACD red cells. The shorter the storage days at +4°C as ACD red cells before freezing, the higher the recovery rate.

MATSUDA et al. (1968) have reported that the recipient's intravascular environment, especially in the presence of certain immunologic, chemical and mechanical factors, largely determines the mean life span of preserved red cells. In our study also the post-transfusion red cell life span of frozen red cells was extremely short in hemolytic anemia-patient as shown in Fig. 40.

Recovery rate and the index of therapeutic effectiveness

Recovery rate : The recovery rate was calculated from the total amount of collected hemoglobin content in the final bag after the entire processing procedure was com-

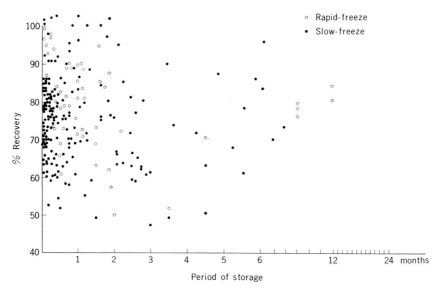

Fig. 42   Percentage recovery of frozen red blood cells after various periods at −80°C and −196°C.

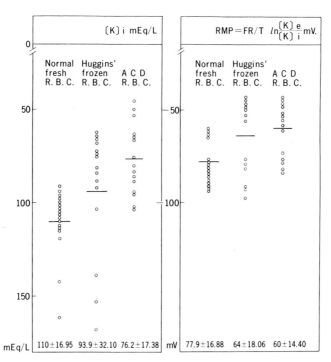

Fig. 43   Intracellular K concentration and resting membrane potential of red blood cells (R.B.C.). Fresh R.B.C. just after collection, frozen R.B.C. frozed for a week at −80°C by slow-freeze, ACD R.B.C. preserved at +4°C for a week.

pleted. Therefore, the hemoglobin concentration and the volume of packed cells before and after the processing were required in order to determine the recovery rate. Since an accurate volume measurement could not be obtained, the volume of the packed red cells was replaced by the weight. Strictly speaking, some error was introduced because the specific gravities of the red cells showed slight difference before and after the processing. The specific gravity was about 1.090 before processing and about 1.106 after processing. These two values were considered to be almost the same, and the following formula was used to calculate the recovery rate of the frozen red cells:

Recovery rate (%)=

$$\frac{\text{Hemoglobin concentration of final bag} \times \text{red cell volume of final bag}}{\text{Hemoglobin concentration of initial bag} \times \text{red cell volume of initial bag}} \times 100$$

The recovery rate was 72.8 ± 10 (n = 50) % in the standard slow-freeze procedure, and 82.9 ± 12.5 (n = 50)% in the rapid-freeze procedure (Figs. 43, 44, and Table 2).

Since April, 1972, we have been using LACTATED-RINGER's solution instead of 0.9% saline for resuspension wash at the final step of the slow-freeze procedure. The recovery rate has increased from 73% to 80%, as shown in Table 4, and the supernatant free hemoglobin concentration to be decanted has decreased remarkably. The explanation for these changes is that LACTATED-RINGER's solution is more physiological than 0.9% saline and contains potassium.

Table 4 Percentage recovery of frozen red cells resuspended by by LACTATED-RINGER's solution.

Resuspension medium	Supernatant hemoglobin concentration		Percentage recovery
	First wash	Second wash	
0.9% saline	889 ± 46 (n=47)	303 ± 53 (n=47)	72.8 ± 10.4 (n=50)
LACTATED-RINGER	635 ± 180 (n= 5)	266 ± 150 (n= 5)	79.9 ± 14.0 (n=65)

The index of therapeutic effectiveness proposed by Valeri (1969): The therapeutic effectiveness-index defines percentage of originally collected donor red cells that have a potential for normal long-term survival in a recipient. This index is determined by multiplication of the *in vitro* recovery value of the cell by the 24-hour post-transfusion survival of the recovered red cells. The index was 70% in the slow-freeze procedure, and 77% in the rapid-freeze porcedure.

ATP content of red cells

The erythrocytes must function in the circulation at the time of transfusion. The preserved red cells at the time of transfusion should have normal levels of organic phosphate compounds (ATP and 2,3-DPG) and normal oxyhemoglobin dissociation characteristics. Adenosintriphosphate (ATP) was measured as an index of the function of freeze-preserved red cells in our clinical study.

Adenosintriphosphate was measured by use of the following principle:

$$ATP = 3\text{-phosphoglycerate} \xrightarrow{\text{PKG}} ADP + 1, 3\text{-diphosphoglycerate}$$

$$1, 3\text{-diphosphoglycerate} + DPNH \xrightarrow{\text{GAPD}} \text{glyceraldehyde-3 phosphate} + DPN + P$$

One ml of blood (heparinized) was added to 1.0 ml of 12% trichloroacetic acid mixed well. It was then allowed to stand for approximately 5 minutes in an ice bath. The centrifuge tube was centrifuged for approximately 5 minutes at about 3000 rpm in order to obtain clear supernatant, 0.5 ml of which were pipetted into a 0.3 mg β-DPNH vial followed by 1.0 ml PGA buffered solution and 1.5 ml water. The vial was inverted several times to dissolve its contents, which were poured into a cuvette of 1 cm light path. The optical density was read and recorded using water as reference at 340 mμ. This was recorded as the initial optical density. 0.04 ml of GAPD/PGK reagent were pipetted into the cuvette, which was inverted and mixed.

The cuvette was replaced in the spectrophotometer. The optical density was read and recorded using water as a reference. The minimum optical density was reached in about 10 minutes, and was recorded as the final optical density. Initial optical density minus final optical density was Δ optical density.

$$\mu \text{ moles of ATP per ml of original sample} = \frac{\Delta OD}{6.22} \times 3.0 \times 4.0 = \Delta OD \times 1.90$$

ATP content of fresh red cells was 2.57 ± 0.32 (n = 20) μmol per gram Hemoglobin, that of the slow-freeze procedures was 1.86 ± 0.55 (n = 32) μmol per gram Hemoglobin, and that of the rapid-freeze procedure was 2.04 ± 0.32 (n = 31) μmol per gram Hemoglobin, as shown in Figs. 30, 31, 32, and Table 2.

Osmotic fragility

In order to avoid misjudgement, the processed red cells should be washed at least three more times with 0.9% saline solution before measurement of the osmotic fragility of frozen red cells. The author's results were 0.49 ± 0.014 (n = 5) of the minimum and 0.44 ± 0.002 (n = 5) of the maximum.

Intracellular potassium concentration and resting membrane potential of frozen red cells

First, the potassium concentration of the supernatant of frozen red cells was measured. The red cells were hemolyzed with the addition of distilled water, and the potassium concentration of the hemolyzed solution was measured. The resting membrane potential was then calculated by NERNST's formula, as shown in Fig. 43. The fresh red cells showed the highest concentration of intracellular potassium, and the ACD red cells preserved for 3 weeks at +4°C showed the lowest. The resting membrane potential was also the highest in the fresh red cells and the lowest in the ACD red cells at the third week. The frozen cells showed the intermediates in the intracellular concentration of potassium and also in the resting membrane potential.

In consideration of the above-mentioned results, we concluded that the membrane permeability of the frozen and the ACD red cells was dependent on the passive rather than the active transport of the membrane and would be easily affected by extracellular fluid changes, with endosmosis occurring in those cells with abnormally decreased potentials. STRUMIA (1966) also determined the potassium and sodium contents of red cells subjected to freezing with 16% dextran by flame photometry. The content of potassium showed a 50% loss, but there was a significant increase in sodium. However, *in vivo* restoration of reversibly damaged liquid-stored or previously frozen red cells have also been demonstrated (CRAWFORD et al., 1955, BEUTLER et al., 1969). The preserved red cells are restored during circulation, suggesting that a satisfactory freeze-preservation procedure must maintain normal intracellular level of sodium and potassium ion, and normal osmotic fragility.

TRANSFUSION AND ITS SIDE EFFECTS, INCLUDING HEPATITIS

Development of capability and flexibility of the blood banking system

Voluntary donations generally decrease in August, Christmas and New Year Season (Fig. 44). It is very difficult to adjust the irregularity of seasonal changes of voluntary blood donations, since the demand for blood is increasing year by year. There also is no idea how post-transfusion serum hepatitis can be prevented except through severe selection of voluntary donors. The author dealt with frozen blood, which can be preserved semi-permanently and purified in each blood component, in order to find a beginning to the resolution of these problems. Medical officials from the United States of America extended the use of frozen blood to the battle line of Vietnam, be-

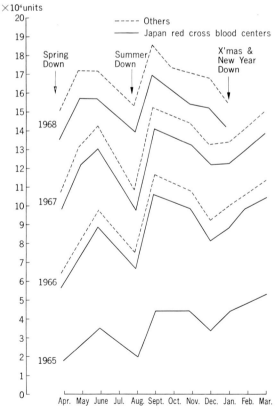

Fig. 44   Voluntary donation of blood in Japan.

cause they could not increase the efficiency of the blood banking system without the use of frozen blood. The unused bloods collected during seasons of sufficient blood donations were freeze-preserved, and they were used during the seasons when there was a shortage of blood donations. By these means, 63 emergency cases were supplied with 299 units of frozen red cells with life saving results (Table 7).

Savings of the blood to be diverted

Bloods with the high GOT (glutaminoxaloacetic transaminase) values over 40, chyle-mia, hemoglobinemia, and syphilis have usually been discarded or diverted as pharma-ceutical raw materials. These bloods could not be utilized as ACD bloods for trans-fusion, even though they were donated by the volunteers' good-will. Those bloods occupied 8.3% of the total amount of donations, of which those having GOT values

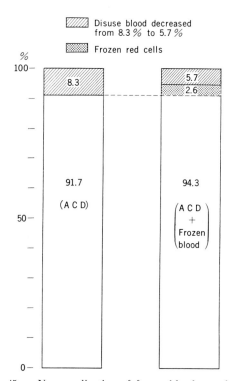

Fig. 45   New application of frozen blood transfusion.

between 40 to 60, and the chyle blood were processed for the frozen red cells, and the percentage of blood to be diverted decreased to 5.7%. Therefore, 2.6% of the whole donated bloods were saved and effectively used for transfusion. According to this method, the frozen red cells were applied for transfusion after washing out of virus and the other plasma components by the deglycerolization process, and this is the "New Application of the Frozen Red Cells" (Fig. 45).

Use of frozen blood for patients with positive transfusion reactions

There were few transfusion reactions to frozen blood owing to the purification of the red cells during the process. Frozen red cells are purified by removal of plasma, leukocytes and platelets. Therefore, the patients who showed strong reactions of urticaria, chills, fever, hypotension, palpitation and so on by the use of banked ACD bloods gladly accepted the transfusion of frozen red cells. Those patients were certain to spe-

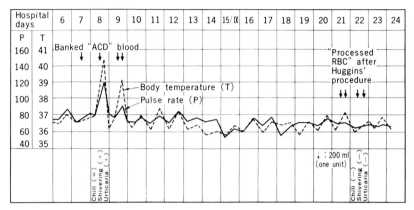

Fig. 46   Frozen red cell transfusion for possitive transfusion reaction.

cifically request frozen blood for future transfusions, and the patients with complaints of chronic and repeated anemia from renal insufficiency and aplastic anemia. The number of transfusions for those patients is now increasing in the National Fukuoka Central Hospital (Fig. 46).

Banking of rare type of blood for autotransfusion and for scientific materials

Like planned pregnancy and delivery, blood banking can also be planned ahead through the technique of frozen blood. Just before their marriages women are especially urged to donate and preserve their blood for themselves. This is a minor application of the technique for the indefinite storage of blood from an individual in health, for readministration as autologous blood at a later date. Unfortunately, a certain religious sect (JEHOVAH's Witnesses) occasionally do not accept this advantage on religious grounds (PERRAULT, 1967), but ROWE (1969) has reported that this religious sect has agreed to receive their own frozen blood. Recently, two patients having Rh negative blood types were saved by frozen blood transfusions because of the shortage of a rare type of blood in Fukuoka City. One of these patients was in deep shock with atonic bleeding after delivery, and the other was a case of unexpected bleeding during abdominal surgery. Those rare types of blood had been preserved for 2 years, because some patients having Rh negative blood stockpiled many units of blood for their operations, and their operations did not require the use of the collected bloods, which had been separated into red blood cells and plasma, and the red cells had been frozen. Thus if one has his blood frozen when he is healthy, he can use his own blood if an emergency occurs. There will be no possibility of contraction of post-transfusion hepatitis. As a result of these advantages, programmed blood banking is increasing in our hospital.

It is impossible to execute the preservation of the rare types of blood and variable blood for scientific materials without freeze preservation. The autobanking of those types of blood started at the frozen blood section of the National Fukuoka Central Hospital in May, 1969, by collecting the bloods by erythrocytpheresis from the donors who have the blood type of Rh null and so on. These "uncommon" bloods (O, Rh negative) could be used as universal donor bloods in emergency with a higher margin of safety in Japan. If these rare types are not used for the donors themselves, they can be used for their descendants. One of the manufactures of low temperature equipment in the United States of America is propagating the freeze preservation of blood by the catch-phrase, "The blood you give today could save your great-great grandson's life". The studies on frozen blood, although originally undertaken in response to military demands in the United States of America, have yielded information that can prove to be equally valuable in civilian situations.

Uses of frozen blood for patients with kidney and heart insufficiency

As the antigens of leukocyte and platelets are not confirmed as well as those of red cells, cross matching of those cells are not usually performed in the present status. Transfusion reactions of chills and urticaria were provoked in the patients who received transfusions, because of antibody formation for foreign leukocytes and platelets, when the dialyzer was primed with banked ACD bloods.

Usually these nonhemolytic transfusion reactions are either given little consideration or neglected, but they are troublesome for patients. These reactions will undoubtedly be taken into consideration when artificial dialysis and organ transplantation become more popular. It should also be noted that frozen blood is plasma free and contains very few leukocytes, and platelets, which are destroyed during the freezing process. Even patients who previously complained of fever, lethargy and urticaria will not show any complications by the use of frozen blood. Frozen red cells can be suspended in 5% albumin solution for the same purpose. These clinical indications of frozen red cells for those patients in whom the formations of antibodies for leukocytes and platelets are undoubtedly considered, will be widely expanded in the near future. HUGGINS, C. E. (1964, 1966) has used frozen blood transfusions for such patients in order to prevent the second-set-like rejection after organ transplantations. He used deglycerolized red cells as white-blood-cell deficient blood for patients sensitized to leukocytes and for patients undergoing chronic dialysis, as well as for pre-, intra-, and post-operative transfusion of renal allotransplant recipients. More than 1000 units of frozen red cells have been given to those patients. He expected that removal of the white cells by selective destruction during the freeze-thaw-wash process virtually eliminated the problem of "reactions" in patients sensitized to leukocytes. Frozen blood has a low supernatant potassium concentration (Table 3), which is more favourable than the use of the banked ACD blood for patients with renal and cardiac insufficiency. Potassium is transported into the extracellular space outside the red-cell wall when red cells are preserved in the ACD solution at 4°C because of unsatisfactory conditions for red cell metabolism. The supernatant potassium concentration of the ACD blood was 12 mEq per L at the 7th day after collection, 17 at the 14th day and 20 at the 21st day (STRUMIA, 1963). When red cells are transfused or rewarmed to body temperature, potassium is retransported into the cells. However, those high con-

Table 5 Extracorporeal hemodialysis with frozen red cells.

No.	Sex/Age	Diagnosis			Na	K	Cl	U-N	pH	PO$_2$	PCO$_2$	O$_2$Sat.	S.B.	B.B.	B.E	Hours of dialysis
1	♂/46	Renal tuberculosis	1st time	pre-	132.2	6.2	106.2	116.0								2
				post-	138.0	4.9	105.8	49.9								
2	♂/61	Gastric cancer postop.	1st time	pre-	141.8	5.9	93.0	109.5								2.5
				post-	136.0	5.2	93.0	97.5								
3	♀/25	Mercury intoxication	1st time	pre-	140.0	5.7	93.1	133.5	7.10	178	20.0					3
				post-	146.5	3.2	115.3	29.0	7.07	101	22.0	90.8				
			2nd time	pre-	140.0	6.5	96.1	179.0	7.102	78	21.0	88.8				3
				post-	151.0	3.2	119.8	29.5	7.180	85	25.2	92.5				
4	♂/29	Postoperative acute renal failure	1st time	pre-	140.0	5.5	92.5	190.8	7.368	85	29.5	95.3	19.0	43.3	− 6.8	4
				post-	143.5	4.0	120.8	54.0	7.470	113	29.5	97.3	22.5	44.5	− 1.8	
			2nd time	pre-	140.0	6.3	95.0	327.0	7.240	106	25.0	96.3	13.3	33.2	−15.5	3
				post-	144.5	5.7	103.0	276.1	7.369	122	20.2	98.2	16.1	39.8	−11.1	
			3rd time	pre-	140.5	7.25	100.0	325.6	7.340	45	16.3	74	9.6	33.7	−16.8	4
				post-	132.0	6.35	99.0	291.0	7.375	64	10↓	89.2	10.5	26.4	−18.8	

centrations of potassium in the supernatant will of course be harmful for the patients of uremia, acute renal failure and severe burns, even if it is temporary. HAYNES (TULLIS, 1966) reported that the potassium concentration of serum decreased from 7.82 mEq to 6.82 mEq per L and electrocardiogram was improved after the transfusion of packed red cells washed with a medium without potassium. The author also tried artificial dialyses by use of frozen red cells for five patients with renal tuberculosis, chronic renal failure, and acute renal failure from bichlolide of mercury and so on,

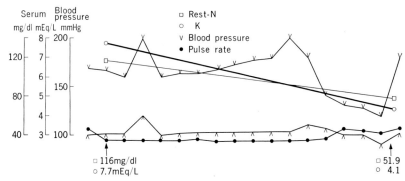

Fig. 47   Extracorporeal hemodialysis by frozen red cells priming (Case No. 1).

and got good results (Fig. 47, and Table 5). The supernatant of frozen blood has a low concentration of potassium, and the frozen blood neither contains sodium citrate nor vasoactive substances of plasma. Therefore, frozen blood transfusion is well indicated for patients with hemorrhagic diathesis from acute renal failure and for patients with heart failure and abnormally increased extracellular fluid.

Frozen blood component therapy

We cannot obtain a variety of blood products from the pharmaceutical companies at present, and it may not be possible to handle frozen blood cells except plasma fractions of albumin, globulin, cryoprecipitate, and others. This is because it is rather difficult to master the technique of the processing of frozen blood cells and there is no settled criterion for guarantee of the product. Therefore, the freeze preservation of blood cells (i.e., red cells, platelets, white cells and bone marrows), will be processed at special institutes and hospitals for a considerable period hereafter. Red cells, platelets, bone marrow and cryoprecipitate are preserved in the frozen state as frozen blood components in our frozen blood section. Platelets are first separated from the ACD blood just after collection and then frozen, and the platelet-poor plasma is immediately reinfused to the donor. The red cells are frozen by the previously mentioned procedure. If the donor refuses the erythrocytpheresis, the platelet-poor plasma is used to separate cryoprecipitate (the Factor VIII) and other fractions.

The frozen blood component therapy allowed separation and storage of a variety of blood components, and their recombination when needed in specific clinical situations.

Demand for frozen blood

Compared with ACD blood, frozen blood transfusion is a little more complicated in the post-thaw processing, but it has many merits, as shown in Table 6. Frozen blood is more expensive than the ACD and CPD blood. However, the cost will be minimized when the other blood components are utilized more widely. Transfusion of frozen red cells is indicated for the diseases shown in Table 6 based on experience of HUGGINS, C. E. (1965). In the National Fukuoka Central Hospital having 500 beds, the transfusion of frozen red cells unexpectedly increased to about 80–100 units per

Table 6 Merits of frozen red cell transfusion.

1. "Long term preservation" produces:
   No out-dated blood,
   Immediate availability of rare blood,
   Blood for autogenous use

2. "Purification" produces:
   Low potassium content (convenient for renal failure, heart failure),
   Markedly reduced leukocyte count (no urticaria, chill, or shivering),
   No platelets (same as above),
   No protein or allergens (same as above),
   No anticoagulant (no bleeding tendency or citrate intoxication),
   Few anti-A and anti-B isoagglutinins in group 0 red cells (universal donation)

3. Low incidence of serum hepatitis

month, occupying about 30% of the total units used in the hospital. VALERI (1968 b) reported that 7% of all blood transfused at the Massachusetts General Hospital, Boston were in the form of HUGGINS' processed red cell. About 10% of the frozen blood processed in our frozen blood section were used in the other hospitals, mainly at the Kyushu University Hospital and sometimes used outside of Fukuoka Prefecture. Frozen blood was transfused to those patients shown in Table 7. It would not be long before frozen blood becomes one of the standard necessities of the hospitals in Japan.

Table 7 Frozen blood transfusion (1969. 1. /1973. 2. 28).

	No. of recipients	No. of frozen blood units
1. Shortage	215 (55 %)	1546
2. Anemia	67 (17 %)	428
3. Emergency	63 (16 %)	299
4. Transfusion reaction	9 (2 %)	228
5. Hepatic failure	16 (4 %)	189
6. Renal failure	16 (4 %)	210
7. Rh negative	3 (1 %)	8
8. Others	1 (0.3%)	26
Total No.	391	2934

(Two patients and 31 units were not investigated)

Criteria for frozen blood transfusion

As previously mentioned, HUGGINS' procedure was modified and standardized by the author in Japan.   However, VALERI (1969, 1970) reported recently that the preservation period of red blood cells by HUGGINS' method would be limited to 1–1.5 years, because this technique uses the cryoprotective solution with low ionic and high glycerol concentration.   When a longer preservation of red cells is required the slow-freeze procedure with cryoprotective solution containing much more electrolyte and glycerol or the rapid-freeze procedure with electrolyte and low glycerol solution should be adopted.   ROWE (1968, 1969) transfused 1000 units of the rapid-freeze red blood cells preserved in liquid nitrogen vapor at −150°C protected with glycerol solution of low concentration.   The deglycerolization was done by batch-wash.   This rapid-freeze procedure was originally devised by PERT et al. (1963) and was further developed by KRIJNEN et al. (1965, 1968) and ROWE (1968, 1969).   They respectively applied their unique containers and constitutions of cryoprotective solutions as previously mentioned.   PERT used sucrose-glycerol solution and Teflon container, ROWE mannitol-glycerol solution and stainless steel container (and recently cryogenically stable plastic bag), KRIJNEN sorbitol-glycerol and aluminum bottle, and VINOGRAD-FINKEL et al. (1971) also used mannitol-glycerol and aluminum corrugated container in each situation.

In New York, ROWE has by far the greatest experience with these of rapid-freeze blood.   The author is also using the stainless steel containers originated by ROWE (Fig. 34) and his cryoprotective solution of low concentration of glycerol.   One hundred and ninety-four units of rapid-freeze red blood cells were transfused into 64 patients in our hospital.   The clinical results seemed satisfactory.   When the complicated and somewhat hazardous procedure are improved, this technique will undoubtedly be the most popular.   The National Research Council National Academy of Science Committee on Blood and Transfusion Problems of the United States of America has proposed guidelines in order to evaluate the results of various freeze-preservation methods in civilian and military medical practice.   The Committee divided the uses of frozen red cells into two major groups: (a) the limited requirements for blood transfusion in special circumstances—rare red blood cells, autologous transfusions, surgical procedures requiring large quantities of blood, and (b) the circumstances in which ACD blood is usually given (VALERI, 1969 a, b).   However, if frozen blood were to be used more often in place of the ACD blood, several problems would arise which should be improved immediately; such as the hazardous technique, the expensive price, and the technical loss of red blood cells.   Apart from the considerations of operational effort and expense, if frozen blood is to be used as a substitute for ACD blood on equal clinical terms, the frozen product should meet the following biological requirements (VALERI, 1969 b).

(1)   Total loss of red blood cells 24 hours after transfusion not be greater than those in the transfusion of ACD blood as specified by National Institute of Health (NIH) Regulations.   In addition, the decline of the red blood cells population surviving the first 24 hours after transfusion should be similar to that of normal red blood cells.

(2)   Preserved blood should not contain any additive that is toxic in man, that is not rapidly excreted or metabolized, or that is likely to sensitize the patient by reason of an antigenic component.

(3) The preserved cells should be stable at low temperatures for at least one year, as measured by standard red blood cells survival studies.

(4) Immediately and for at least 72 hours after thawing, red blood cells that have been stored in the frozen state should possess, as a minimum, physiological and bacteriological attributes similar to those of 21-day-old ACD blood stored under regular blood bank conditions.

(5) The immediate and long-term condition of the recipient's health should not be prejudiced by any untoward secondary effect from a single or large multiple transfusion of preserved blood.

(6) If possible, red blood cells should be packaged so as to permit the use of the same container for collecting, freezing, storing, thawing, and transfusing. This is particularly important to ensure maintenance of donor identification. In any event, however, the container used during the transfusion should permit direct visual inspection of the blood.

We believe that our blood freezing technique will satisfy these criteria. The frozen red cells might be used more widely for anemic patients who need packed red cells. In our hospital the frozen red cells are now used by the patients' own accord under more extensive indications. Frozen blood is ready to be used at a moment's notice for transfusion. That is a boon to emergency cases. Therefore, we should not hesitate to accept the above-mentioned complicated criteria, otherwise we will lose sight of the merits of frozen blood transfusions. We certainly believe that frozen red cell transfusions promote an interest and the popularization of the concept of blood component therapy in Japan.

Frozen blood and post-transfusion serum hepatitis

The prevention of hepatitis after blood transfusion has been one of the most elusive problems of blood banking, because there is no absolute method of detecting the hepatitis carrier among blood donors. Huggins (1965, 1969) introduced the frozen blood transfusion to Japan at the 13th Annual Meeting of the Japanese Society of Blood Transfusion (President Prof. Shuichi Hayashi) in 1965, where he gave a noteworthy report that administration of previously frozen blood had apparently not been followed by clinical viral hepatitis, and that the freezing process may lower the infectivity of virus or the post-thawing process may dilute and wash out the virus. The author, as well as the audience, was deeply impressed by Huggins' speech about the incidence of serum hepatitis. At the same time, a question remained, that being whether the virus was inactivated by freezing at $-85°C$ or completely washed out. The following are the advantages of transfusion of frozen red cells: (a) the low isoagglutinin titer of resuspended frozen blood is helpful in that all patients may be given Group O blood, matching only the Rh type to that of the recipient (Table 3), (b) one can eliminate citrate anti-coagulants, and minimize the potassium content of blood for transfusion, (c) urticarial reactions are eliminated, (d) white blood cells are removed by deglycerolization wash, meaning removal of formed elements other than the donors' erythrocytes (Fig. 38), and (e) blood can be stored for long periods. However, the above-mentioned advantages, except the long-term storage and purification of blood cells, are essentially the same as those of washed red cells. The fact that there was no incidence of post-transfusion hepatitis cannot be directly related to the inactivation of virus by the physical process of freezing at −85°C to −80°C, as already mentioned by Huggins (1965, 1966).

The virus of hepatitis is indeed a virulence with a strong resistance against the circumstances of freezing and also against glycerol. Virus can usually be preserved at sub-zero temperatures down to −80°C to −196°C after addition of high concentrations of glycerol: therefore, it cannot be considered that virus is inactivated at those temperatures. One should be inclined to consider that virus is preserved, of course, alive in the glycerol solution. For these reasons, the procedure itself probably has an important significance concerning the low incidence of post-transfusion serum hepatitis. It was a hasty conclusion to make following Huggins' report that no serum hepatitis was produced by the transfusion if the red blood cells having hepatitis virulence were processed as frozen blood. There is no reliable procedure to inactivate hepatitis virus from the clinical point of view. Neither ultraviolet irradiation, betapropiolactone, high energy ^{60}Co gamma irradiation, pans No. 610, nor sodium monochloroacetate were entirely successful for the inactivation of the virus. Therefore, one must conclude that the inactivation of serum hepatitis will be difficult indeed. Recently we tried administration of gamma-globulin, which also resulted in imperfect prevention of the disease. In short, there are two preventive measures against serum hepatitis; first, the purification with physiochemical processing of red cells, and second, the careful selection of donors with their anamnesis and the serological test as well as Australia antigen test. As frozen red cells are washed several times in a large volume of sugar solution and/or salt solution during the deglycerolization process, during which plasma components and hepatitis virus might be excluded. However, the perfect purification of red cells was extremely difficult, and we feel that the imperfect purification by washing might be technically impossible. Miura (1969) indirectly suggested an *in vivo* experiment with poliovirus Type I, New Castle disease virus, Coliphage T_3W, and Coliphage 174 that removal of the plasma and washing of red blood cells with sugar solutions utilizing his own design of a cytoglomerator may eliminate the possibility of transmitting homologous serum hepatitis. Therefore, we could not continue frozen blood transfusion without any consideration of hepatitis risk. The incidence rate of post-transfusion serum hepatitis from frozen blood transfusion is currently very slight, but the situation does not warrant optimism. It is very dangerous and optimistic to think that we have no problem with frozen blood as far as prevention of serum hepatitis and blood transfusion reaction are concerned. Recently, Huggins, C. E. (1972) reported a case of post-transfusion serum hepatitis from frozen red cells at the Massachusetts General Hospital.

A combination of careful donor selection, meticulous reporting of all cases of hepatitis, routine testing for Australia antigen, and the judicious use of blood and blood products including frozen red cells should prevent many cases of post-transfusion hepatitis, of which judicious use of blood is the most important factor. Blood and blood components should be used only when truly indicated. The single-unit transfusion should be used with great caution and should be avoided unless absolutely necessary. All component therapy as previously mentioned and frozen blood transfusion should be evaluated with as much care as that used for whole-blood transfusion. Considering the above-mentioned results, we cannot help reaching the conclusion that there is no direct relationship between the clinical use of frozen red cells and the prevention of serum hepatitis. The advantage of frozen blood may be just a long-termed preservation of blood cells. HUGGINS reported that he had never experienced serum hepatitis after frozen blood transfusion, which led us to believe that there was no serum hepatitis produced by frozen blood transfusion. It was one of our biggest objects to confirm his results. By February, 1966, HUGGINS (1969) had transfused 2229 units of frozen red blood cells, which produced no post-transfusion hepatitis. He also mentioned that there was no statistically significant difference in the incidence rate of serum hepatitis between frozen blood and banked ACD blood, and he explained that hepatitis virus would be washed out during deglycerolization with a large volume of sugar solution. Considering that inactivation of the virus would be impossible by freezing, we had expected the same results as HUGGINS'. We must bear in mind that we have given a wrong impression not only to the physicians but also to the general public in Japan that frozen blood did not produce post-transfusion hepatitis.

Table 8   Occurrence of icteric serum hepatitis by frozen blood and ACD blood.

	Total donations	No. of patients	No. of instances of hepatitis	Percent
Tokyo 1965/1968	290 frozen blood only	82	1	1.2
Kyushu 1969/1972	1246 frozen blood only	267	6	2.2
	722 frozen blood+ACD blood	94	7	7.4

(Thirty patients were not investigated.)

Recently, WERCH et al. (1971) reported an interesting paper on detection of Australia antigen in various fractions of frozen blood. Their results with frozen blood revealed that HUGGINS' procedure of freezing, thawing, and washing was associated with loss of detectable Au/SH antigen in six of the seven erythrocyte samples, accounting for the observation that clinical post-transfusion hepatitis has not occurred after administration of frozen blood. Judging from the results of our frozen blood transfusion for 7 years in Japan, as shown in Table 8, we cannot eliminate serum hepatitis from frozen blood transfusion.

Disadvantages and side effects

Transient hemoglobinemia: Table 9 shows side effects from frozen blood transfusion for the past 3 years. There were no descriptions on post-transfusion hemoglobinemia from frozen blood in the papers by HUGGINS, C. E. (1964, 1965a, b, 1966). He described frozen blood as resembling packed red cells. We have used frozen red cell transfusion since October, 1965, and have continuously discussed transient post-transfusion hemoglobinemia and serum hepatitis. When we began transfusing frozen blood, we experienced three cases of hemoglobinemia out of 64 patients who received frozen blood. One case produced a hemoglobinemia of 500 ml per dl hemoglobin concentration after 5 units of frozen blood were transfused, and the other showed wine-red urine. The serum free hemoglobin concentration of these patient was about 150 mg per dl just after transfusion, and the other patient showed a remarkable hemoglobinemia.   Ahaptoglobinemia was not confirmed by electrophoresis in these three patients who showed hemoglobinemia.   We reached the conclusion that frozen red cells transfused into the patient would be totally hemolyzed *in vivo*.   The causes of those massive hemolyses were considered as follows: (a) the glass bottles having a limited volume (Fig. 48), which were used previously for the freeze preservation and were not big enough to hold the sufficient volume of 79% glycerol solution to be added to the

Table 9   Side effects of frozen blood transfusion.

Chill and fever	8
Hemoglobinuria	3
Urticaria	3
Local vascular pain	1
Abdominal pain	1
Fatigue	1
Hypotension	1
Total	18

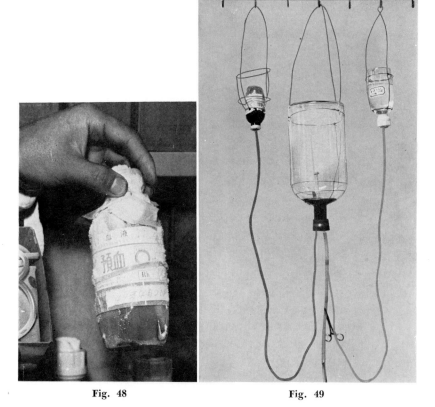

Fig. 48   Fig. 49

Fig. 48   Freeze preservation of red cells in a transfusion glass bottle, produced hemoglobinuria.

Fig. 49   Deglycerolization glass bottle (SUMIDA, 1965).

packed red cells for cryoprotection, (b) 2.0% saline solution was used for resuspension of the several units of frozen red cells, and the red cells shrunk from hypertonicity of 2.0% saline, resulting in hemolysis *in vivo* from the mechanism of osmotic shock, (c) the ACD red cells used for frozen red cells at the 16th to 20th day after collection, and their osmotic competencies were too fragile to freeze them, (d) deglycerolization was not perfect because of the usage of a large washing bottle (Fig. 49). PERRAULT (1967) transfused 101 units of frozen red cells into 12 patients with leukemia, and one of these patients produced hemoglobinuria. This case was not the patient with ahaptogloblinemia. He reported that the other patient with ahaptoglobinemia showed hemoglobinuria. There was a moderate decrease in haptoglobin concentration, the maximum reduction being 190 mg% (from 470 to 280). At the same time, hemoglobinemia appeared in Vietnam combat casualities from massive transfusion of frozen red cells (Moss et al., 1966, 1968).

This transient hemoglobinuria after frozen blood transfusion is one of the most unpleasant and dangerous side effects for the patients. After taking a considerable amount of time and effort to eliminate it, the following criteria were settled upon as the principal solution: (a) packed ACD red cells should be used for the frozen red cells within 7 days after collection, (b) the same volume of 79% glycerol solution should be added to the packed red cells allowing at least 15 minutes or more to mix well, (c) the same volume of 50% glucose solution for deglycerolization after thawing should slowly be added into the thawed glycerolized red cells, (d) resuspension wash in 0.9% saline solution should preferably be repeated twice, in order to wash out the supernatant free hemoglobin as much as possible. There were no fatal side effects but there was the above-mentioned transient hemoglobinuria.

Price of frozen red cells: Owing to the high price of frozen red cells, they are not widely popularized. PERRAULT (1967) in Canada reported that the cost of one unit of processed frozen blood was $20, which included only the special bag and the cost of wash solution, but neither the cost of HUGGINS' cytoglomerator at $10,000 nor the deep-freezers at a minimum of about $3,300. We are now supplying a unit of frozen red cells at ¥7150 (about $24) in Japan, which includes the cost of a plastic container (SUMIDA's blood freezing unit), the cryoprotective and wash solutions, and the cost of maintenance and personal expenditures. We do believe that the cost will be remarkably reduced if frozen blood component therapy develope in a way that blood centers supply each component at sufficient cost to offset the slight added cost of frozen blood.

Frozen blood and protein deficiency: Frozen red cells are usually resuspended by 0.9% saline which does not contain protein. TULLIS (1966) resuspended frozen red cells in 5% albumin solution. If we use only the packed red cells for transfusion, but this does not always mean that the packed red cell transfusion has no efficacy to treat the low proteinemia. CALLOWAY (1953) reported that serum portein increased from 4 g to 7 g per dl after transfusion of 1250 ml of packed red cells. YOSHINAGA (1958) reported that transfusion of 400 ml to 2,900 ml packed red cells resulted in an increase of serum protein, no tendency to homorrhagic disorder, and good postoperative results. Globin of the red cells contains each amino acid except isoleucine, corresponding 2 times to 3 times as much protein as the serum content. We were very interested in CALLOWAY's conclusion that the synthesis of hemoglobin might be facilitated by red cell transfusion, even if the hemoglobin of transfused red cells was not included in the synthesis of red cell hemoglobin. MURRAY (1943) reported that the transfusion of packed red cells could occupy up to 50% of the total units of blood used in the university hospital. About 30% or more of all transfusion at the National Fukuoka Central Hospital are frozen red cells. It is not a disadvantage, but rather an advantage that the frozen red cells contain neither platelets nor protein. The frozen platelets can also be thawed and used anytime when needed. Whole blood should be primarily required for the maintenance of effective circulating blood volume, which is reduced in acute hemorrhage or in shock due to violence, burns or infection.

3

Platelets

FROZEN PLATELETS AND THEIR HISTORICAL REVIEW

At the present time we have excellent evidence of long term preservation of erythro-cytes in glycerol as previously mentioned. The application to granulocytes is also suc-cessful in regard to human studies.

In a sense it may be said that the platelets are one of the most important blood com-ponents to be preserved in the frozen state. Under the law of biological standard for blood banking, it is well known that platelets are largely destroyed in ACD solution after being preserved at a temperature of 4°C for 5 days. Therefore, the platelets col-lected as ACD blood by voluntary donation are discarded as cell debris. Once frozen platelet transfusions become technically available, the demands will eventually increase remarkably. Platelet transfusions are indicated for idiopathic thrombocytopenic pur-pura and iatrogenic thrombocytopenia during treatment of malignancies. REBUCK (1963) reported that viable platelet levels in ACD banked blood stored at 4°C fall appreciably after 3 hours of such storage and then fall precipitously after 24 hours of storage. The maximum storage period of platelet-rich plasma removed from whole blood is approximately 10 hours, while that of platelet concentrates is 4 hours, based on a loss of less than 50% of transfused platelets. Platelets stored at 4°C have been found to lose their ability to survive after transfusion in direct proportion to their storage time (KREVANS, 1961). The freeze preservation of platelets is not practical at the present time. Initial studies by TULLIS et al. (1953) indicated that platelets derived from ACD plasma could be suspended in sterile 1.4% gelatin in an acetate saline solution. Platelet then were stored at 4°C for varying number of weeks, during which the preserved platelets were relatively inert metabolically, and showed a sur-vival period of 1–3 days in transfused patients. The gelatin-preserved platelets exhibited some clinical effectiveness; the hemostasis was obtained perhaps by auto-catalytic stimulation of new platelet production for temporary correction of a thrombo-plastic deficit (TULLIS et al., 1959). And, such platelets showed excellent preservation of *in vitro* clotting factors for period up to 2 years. However, they have demonstrated only minimal elevations of platelet counts after reinfusion into patients. Studies on preservation of rat platelets in gelatin have given no evidence of such platelets circu-lating in the recipient (FIRKIN et al., 1960, RACCUGLIN et al., 1960).

KLEIN (1956 a) transfused platelets concentrated and preserved in plasma at −15°C for up to 6 weeks for thrombocytopenic patients, resulting in a transitory hemostasis.

However, the evidence showed that platelets preserved at low temperature could control bleeding. KLEIN (1956 b) also administered lyophilized platelet material to children with acute leukemia and aplastic anemia, resulting in some transient hemostasis and some correction of defective prothrombin consumption. After that, FLIEDNER (1958) tested the efficacy of fresh versus lyophilized platelet transfusions in rats to control radiation-induced hemorrhage. While fresh platelet transfusions doubled or tripled the normal count and stopped hemorrhage, the lyophilized material had no effect on count elevation nor on the cessation of bleeding tendency. JACKSON et al., (1958) also found no evidence of hemostatic response following infusion of lyophilized platelets.

Several fundamental and original studies have been done on the preservation of platelets at low temperature by use of cryoprotective additives such as glycerol and DMSO, and the slow freezing methods previously mentioned have been employed with platelets. WEISS and BALLINGER (1958) applied initially the glycerol technique to preserve dog platelets, which were frozen in glycerol and stored for period of up to 4 months at −79°C. The thawed platelets were viable as evidenced by retention of morphological characteristics and clot retracting activity. These studies were later extended to the preservation of human platelets by WEISS and BALLINGER (1958), who examined *in vivo* and *in vitro* survival of glycerolized frozen human platelets and found that survival rate was about 25% of unfrozen controls and occasionally reached 50% to 70% of the controls. COHEN and GARDNER (1959, 1966) have also studied the freeze preservation of canin platelet concentrates obtained from blood anticoagulated with ACD or EDTA were mixed with glycerol to a final concentration of 7.5% to 10% vol./vol. of plasma. They obtained evaluation of various glycerol concentrations and used a final 12% concentration of glycerol. Glycerolized platelet concentrate was cooled at a rate of 1°C per minute until −30°C was reached followed by 5°C per minute until −70°C was reached, and stored for 1 week to 3 weeks. Thereafter, they were rapidly thawed at 7–10°C per minute. The glycerol was washed out with 12% dextrose, and resuspended in platelet-poor plasma. COHEN and GARDNER (1966) also confirmed that the additives of glycerol and dextrose to the platelet concentrate without freezing and thawing did not influence yield of life span of labeled canine platelets. Therefore, there is a large loss of platelets associated with the freezing and thawing.

After the deglycerolization frozen platelets had only a 25% decrease in initial viability in comparison to untreated fresh plasma. This loss of viability was acceptable for a large scale preservation program. Using glycerol freezing techniques and ^{51}Cr labeling for the determination of post-thaw survival, they found 30–35% of the frozen-thawed platelets surviving in human recipients.

BALDINI (1966) had also applied the technique of glycerol freezing to human platelets and his data have been similar to the results mentioned; namely, about 25% yield of glycerol frozen-thawed platelets. These researches for the preservation of canine and human platelets are highly encouraging us. Aside from glycerol, DMSO (dimethylsulfoxide) have been used as a cryoprotective agent by several investigators (IOSSIFIDES et al., 1962, DJERASSI et al., 1964), and the rapid preservation technique with liquid nitrogen have been also tried. A variety of additives has been used, but a final concentration of 5–7% dextrose in a 5% DMSO solution has improved platelet function *in vitro* after freezing and has been the diluent for clinical studies (DJERASSI et al., 1962, 1963).   And, in a study comparing fresh platelet transfusion with frozen platelet concentrates, the increment of the platelet count in thrombocytopenic recipients with frozen platelets was one third the yield obtained with fresh platelets.   That is 31%.

At the Annual Meeting of the Society for Cryobiology at Washington, D.C. in 1971, ROWE reported on the study of differences in human platelets permeability to glycerol and DMSO.   According to ROWE, the change in platelet volume is primarily responsible for the differences observed here between glycerol and DMSO uptake, indicating the presence of a partial barrier to glycerol entry into human platelets.   KIM and BALDINI (1971) conducted studies on the effects of cryoprotective agents and freezing glycolysis and adenine nucleotides of human platelets and concluded that: (a) the increase in glycolytic activity which occurred before freezing in the platelets exposed to cryoprotective agents may be interpreted as a reaction to cellular damage, (b) freezing and thawing produced abrupt depression of platelet glycolysis and reduction of ATP, (c) the smallest changes were observed in platelets treated with DMSO only.

WEATHERBEE et al. (1971) reported on a procedure for storage of Rhesus monkey platelets at $-80°C$ applicable for use with human thrombocytes.   They used acidified ACD solution as an anticoagulant to collect platelets from monkeys by plasmapheresis. Platelet concentrates were prepared by centrifugation at $26°C$ and hydroxyethyl starch (HES) was added to the platelet concentrate.   The final concentration of HES was 6%(w/v).   The platelet-starch mixture was cooled at $37°C$ per minute to $-80°C$ and stored at this temperature for 6–8 days.   The platelets were thawed with agitation in a $47°C$ water bath, then labeled with ^{51}Cr.   Recovery was determined at 2, 24, 48, and 72 hours.   Preliminary results indicated 33–55% survival after 24 hours, and good recovery of platelets after freeze-thaw procedure.

DAYIAN, CHIN and ROWE (1971) extended their study to include the determination of the cooling rates and glycerol concentration most effective in preventing cryoinjury to platelet lysosomes.   The percentage of enzyme release noted with the different concentrations of glycerol (0.1–1.0 M) followed a parallel change throughout the range of cooling rates.   The optimum cooling rate at each glycerol concentration was about $30°C$ per minute while the optimum glycerol concentration at all cooling rates was 0.55 M.   Under optimum cooling rate and glycerol concentration the activation or release of beta-glucuronidase indicated 90–95% of platelet lysosomes remaining intact. ROWE and PETERSON (1971) reported a study of the effect of glycerol, HES, and DMSO on functional integrity of human blood platelets before and after freezing, using ACD platelet-rich plasma and the following parameters: the uptake of ^{14}C-serotonin, the spontaneous release of preadded ^{14}C-serotonin, and the activation of platelet factor-III as measured by Stypven time and platelet aggregation.

After slow ($1°C$ per minute) and moderate ($10–20°C$ per minute) freezing with glycerol 6–8%, DMSO 6–8% and HES 8–10% protection, up to 50% of added serotonin was taken up by the thawed platelets.   Spontaneous release of preadded serotonin was only 20–40% with glycerol and DMSO, although PF-III activity was increased when compared to that of the unfrozen control.   Glycerol at 6–8% would appear to be the most effective cryoprotective additive.   Combinations of glycerol-DMSO and glycerol-HES actually avoided complete release of PF-III after freezing.   ROWE and PETERSON (1971) indicated that combinations of additives proved more effective.   As previously mentioned, much research has been done on the freeze preservation of platelets for several years .

PFISTERER et al. (1969) and DJERASSI et al. (1969) used dimethylacetamide (DMAC) similar to MDSO as an effective cryoprotective additive for rabbit platelets which were frozen at a cooling rate in excess of 100°C per second by direct contact with a surface of liquid helium. The platelets appeared to be almost completely destroyed, however. They then used 5% DMAC in combination with 5% dextrose as a cryoprotective substance for platelet concentrate frozen in liquid nitrogen at a cooling rate of more than 1°C per second. The *in vivo* survival in 30 minutes after transfusion was 75.0% of the control group and 78.2% after 24 hours. Ten % glycerol was significantly less effective than DMAC-dextrose, and appeared less effective than in those specimens in which no additives were used. They also recognized that a warming rate of 40°C per second afforded better protection than that of 6°C per second, in which platelet destruction was heavy. However, there was no description of human platelet preservation. As previously mentioned, the supply of fresh platelet concentrates to thrombocytopenic patients at any time is burdensome for all blood banks, because *in vitro* platelet survival with the present storage technique is too short for practival purpose. Clinical studies mentioned previously would indicate that satisfactory platelet levels could be obtained with frozen platelet for clinical improvement of thrombocytepenia. We initiated research on the preservation technique of human platelets in 1969, using a final 14% concentration of glycerol in a polyvinylchloride plastic bag at a temperature of −80°C.

These concentrates were thawed in a fashion to the previous studies noted above and deglycerolized by adding 13% sodium citrate. Then followed centrifugation and resuspension of the platelet buttom in 0.9% saline or autologous platelet-poor plasma. Two hundred and fifty-four units of frozen platelet concentrate were transfused into 22 patients with idiopathic and iatrogenic thrombocytopenia (Table 10). The platelets frozen by the following procedure were confirmed to have functions of ADP clumping, normal PTT, and clot retraction. A plasma expander, Hydroxyethyl starch (HES), was also proved to preserve platelets in the frozen state, and thus, HES preserved platelets were to be transfused immediately after thawing without the washout process. However, the final constitutions of HES solution as cryoprotectant are now in controversy.

PROCEDURES

Freeze preservation with 28% glycerol solution (SUMIDA, 1970)

Blood was collected as ACD blood from healthy donors in a plastic blood pack, which was centrifuged at approximately 1000 rpm (280 G) for 15 minutes at +22°C. The supernatant plasma containing the platelets was separated and placed in a 300 ml blood transfer pack and then spun again at 3000 rpm (2500 G) for 10 minutes to get platelet concentrate. As the platelets were precipitated at the bottom of the bag, about 60–70 ml of the supernatant plasma were removed and the packed platelets were resuspended in the remaining 30–35 ml of plasma. It was more convenient to process platelet-rich plasma out of six donors to ten donors in one single bag. An equal volume of 28% glycerol solution (ROWE's solution) was added and mixed with the platelet concentrate thus obtained and allowed to

Table 10 Clinical cases of frozen platelets transfusion.

No.	Name	Age/Sex	Blood Type	Diagnosis	Frozen platelets transfusion numbers & donor's hemotype	Pre- and post-transfusion counts of recipient's platelets×10^4	Freeze-preservation period
1	K.H.	45/♂	O	l-pulmonary cancer	4, ① O×4	—	10D× 4
2	T.S.	55/♂	B	r-pulmonary cancer	3, ① B×1, O×2	① 1.4→ 3.8	4～D× 3
3	T.O.	52/♀	A	Gastric cancer	3, ① A×3	② 1.5→ 1.27	3～5D× 3
4	E.K.	38/♀	A	ITP	4, ① A×2, O×2	① 3.0→ 4.2	1～1.5M× 4
5	T.S.	36/♀	AB	ITP	32, ①AB×3 ④AB×4 ②B×3, ⑤AB×5, AB×1 O×5 ③O×5 ⑥AB×5, B×1	① 0.3→ 2.4 ② 0.8→ 5.6 ③～⑥ —	5～6M×10 1～1.5M×10 2–4D× 6
6	R.M.	28/♀	B	ITP	9, ① B×6 ② O×3	—	10D× 2 1～2M× 7
7	I.H.	29/♂	O	KLEINFELTER syndrome	5, ① O×5	① 1.2→ 2.9	
8	K.A.	32/♂	B	Leukemia	14, ① B×6 ② O×8	① 0.8→ 1.6 ② 1.6→ 7.6	5～8M× 4 1～3.5M×10
9	N.K.	14/♀	O	ITP	11, ① O×5 ② O×6	① 3.8→ 1.3 ② 1.3→ 2.0	10M× 5 1M× 6
10	T.H.	66/♂	A	Rectal cancer	11, ① A×11	① 7.8→18.0	1～4M×11
11	M.T.	21/♂	A	ITP	8, ① A×8	—	9M× 5 4～5M× 3
12	M.N.	58/♀	A	ITP	10, ① A×3, O×7	① 6.2→ 3.7	5M× 4 10D× 6
13	Y.O.	44/♂	O	Leukemia & splenomegaly	6, ① O×6	① 27.9→33.5	7M× 1 1M× 2 10D× 3
14	S.Y.	22/♀	AB	ITP	10, ① AB×2, B×8	① 0.3→ 1.3	3.5M× 1 1M× 9
15	H.I.	15/♀	A	ITP	12, ①A×6, O×6	① 3.7→ 2.4	1M×12
16	K.Y.	57/♂	A	ITP	32, ① O×9, A×2 ② A×4, O×7 ③ B×10	—	1M×32
17	K.E.	47/♀	A	Gastric cancer	15, ① B×2, AB×1 ② A×2, O×4 ③ AB×4, O×2	① — ② 6.6→12.4 ③ 12.4→16.7	1M×15
18	H.T.	44/♀	O	Gastric cancer	9, ① A×6, O×3	—	1M× 9
19	H.H.	65/♂	A	Leukemia	9, ① B×2, AB×2 ② O×2, A×1, B×2	① 1.0→ 3.2	1M× 9
20	M.Y.	18/♂	O	Leukemia	18, ① B×8 ② O×10	① 0.4→ 1.6 ② 0.8→ 0.92	1M×18
21	I.O.	68/♂	O	Esophageal cancer	6, ① O×6	—	1M× 6
22	T.I.	62/♂	A	Gastric cancer	23, ① A×10 ② A×9 ③ A×4	—	1M×10 2M×13

Total: 254 units.
Keys : ① means the first transfusion.
B×4 means 4 units of frozen platelets of hemotypĕ B donors.
D means days, M months, × unit-number.

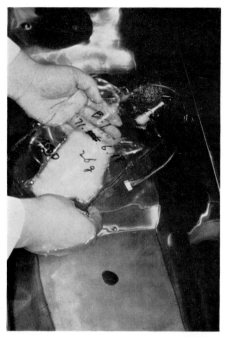

Fig. 50   Thawing of frozen platelets in a water bath at 40°C.

equilibriate for about 10 minutes at +22°C (room temperature) to complete glycerolization.   The plastic bag containing the entire mixture was packaged into a cardboard box and frozen in a deep freezer at −80°C.   Just prior to infusion, the glycerolized frozen platelets were thawed at +45°C in a water bath (Fig. 50), taking about
3 minutes.   Deglycerolization was accomplished by adding 250 ml of 13% sodium
citrate, and the citrate was removed by centrifugation at 3000 rpm (2510 G) for 10 minutes at +22°C.   Frozen platelets were driven to the bottom of the plastic bag as a white
layer (Fig. 51).   The supernatant containing glycerol was decanted, and the same process was repeated once more.   About 30 ml of frozen platelet concentrate remained,

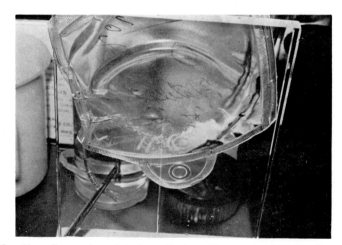

Fig. 51   Frozen-thawed-deglycerolized platelets at the bottom of pack.

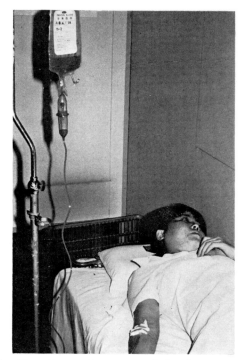

Fig. 52   Frozen platetets transfusion for case no. 15.

which was resuspended by adding 50 ml of 0.9% saline solution.   The original plasma could be used for the resuspension.   The frozen resuspended platelet concentrates were infused into the patients by using an infusion set with a large sized filter, as shown in Fig. 52.   It took about 15 minutes to infuse a whole bag of frozen platelet concentrate.   When a large volume of red cells remained during the process of plasma-pheresis, the frozen platelets were caught at the filter of the infusion set and the infusion was discontinued.   When the freeze preservation of the platelets was not success-ful, the thawed-deglycerolized platelets remained as a solid sediment, which could not

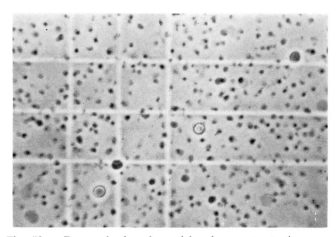

Fig. 53   Frozen platelets observed by phase contrast microscope.

be resuspended by adding 0.9% saline nor by an original plasma. The platelet sediment was observed as a clumping formation under microscopic vision. The maximum preservation period of platelets in the frozen state was 10 months (Table 10).

Freeze preservation with 24% hydroxyethyl starch (Sumida, 1971)

Hydroxyethyl starch (HES) today is in attractive prospect as a cryoprotectant. The HES solution for the cryopreservation of platelets in our frozen blood section contains 24 g of HES, 6 g of mannitol, and 0.65 g of NaCl in 100 ml solution in water. An equal volume of the 24% HES solution was added to the platelet concentrate and well mixed in a plastic bag, which was frozen in a deep freezer at $-80°C$. Just prior to infusion, the plastic bag was plunged into the water bath at a temperature of 45°C and thawed quickly. As HES is a plasma expander as well as a cryoprotectant, the frozen platelet concentrate was immediately infused into the patients without washing out HES after thawing. However, from our clinical experiences, the efficacy of HES as a cryoprotectant for blood cells is now in controversy.

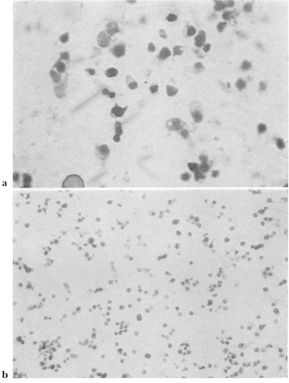

a

b

Fig. 54   Giemsa stained frozen platelets.
Magnification: a×800, b×400.

Pre-transfusion examination of frozen platelets

External appearance of frozen platelet concentrate : Packed frozen platelets were sedimented at the bottom of plastic bag just after the final deglycerolization wash with 13% sodium citrate. The packed frozen platelets were resuspended and homogenized by adding 0.9% saline solution. Shaking and rubbing the bag urged the resuspension of the frozen platelets. When it was difficult to resuspend and homogenize, a lot of fibrin was usually precipitated, making resuspension even more difficult. Even under such circumstances, there were numerous platelets under microscopic vision which could be effectively used for transfusion.

Platelet count of resuspended platelet concentrate : A melangeur for erythrocyte count could be used for counting of frozen platelets after dilution with 14% magnesium sulfate, resulting in 50×10^4–1000×10^4 per mm^3 (Fig. 53). The wide deviations were caused by the processed numbers of platelet-rich plasma in a bag.

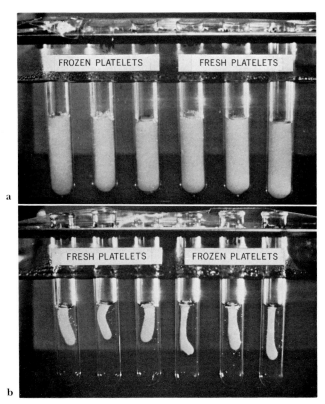

Fig. 55   Clot retraction of fresh and frozen platelets before (a) and after 3 hours (b).

Morphologic observations of frozen platelet smears : Resuspended platelet concentrate films were made on glass slides or coverslips and stained with WRIGHT's stain. Azur granules were seen in a hyaline, light blue cytoplasma. The well preserved platelets were small in size, irregularly shaped and thin-stained. Sometimes much larger platelets were found. Many large, oval, swollen and thick-stained platelets were present, particularly when the preservation was inadequate (Fig. 53).

Clot retraction :   About 0.2 m*l* of resuspended platelet concentrate and a drop of thrombin were added into 0.2% fibrinogen in 0.9% saline in a test tube. This was allowed to remain in a water bath at +37°C and inspected for 3 consecutive hours. Fresh platelets were used as a control (Fig. 55).

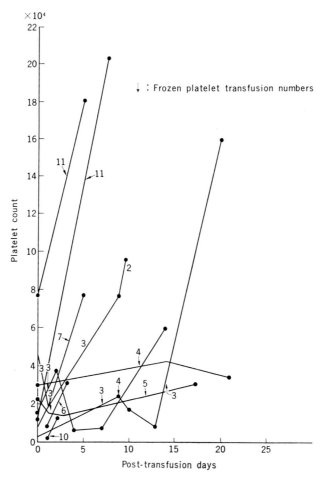

Fig. 56   Changes of platelet counts of recipients.

Post-transfusion examinations of frozen platelets

Platelet count (Fig. 55), bleeding time, coagulation time, and thromboelastogram (Fig. 56 and Table 11) of the recipient were also examined by use of usual techniques of examination. The increase of recipient's platelet count suggests that the frozen platelets are restored during circulation as well as the frozen red cells, and that the frozen platelets stimulate the recipient's hematopoiesis.   However, it was difficult to valuate the true effectiveness of frozen platelet transfusion by clinical cases, because most patient had been simultaneously treated with other drugs.   According to our experience, we had an impression that it was a little difficult to increase the platelet count of patients with idiopathic thrombocytopenic purpura (ITP) by frozen platelet trans-

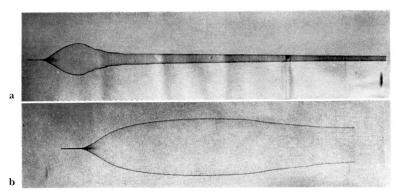

a

b

Fig. 57   Improvement of thromboelastograph of case no. 11. Before frozen platelets transfusion (a) and 24 hours after that (b).

Table   11   Improvement of thromboelastograph before and after
frozen platelet transfusion.

		Before	After
Case No. 10 (M–66)	r	13	11
	k	7	6
	ma	41.5	43
Case No. 11 (M–21)	r	10	10.3
	k	10	9
	ma	32	44

fusion, because the hematopoiesis of the recipient bone marrow might be irreversibly
destroyed or thrombocyte antibody formed by the previous transfusion might have
produced the early destruction of frozen platelets in the recipient's intravascular
environment.

1) Glycerol-Slow

NaCl (w/v %)

NaCl	0	10	20	30	40	50	60	70	80	90
18.0	0	18	13	30	37	34	37	51	86	81
9.0	0	22	12	22	15	21	41	81	90	79
5.0	0	0	0	0	24	40	75	85	79	68
3.2	0	15	5	16	22	46	86	77	91	71
2.4	0	0	0	0	39	90	82	98	93	43
2.2	0	0	0	0	59	96	98	97	91	22
2.0	0	0	0	1	47	87	98	93	83	30
1.8	0	0	0	0	73	91	98	98	96	34
1.6	0	4	4	0	80	96	98	96	94	51
1.4	0	8	0	12	83	97	94	91	68	21
1.2	0	0	1	46	82	96	97	85	40	8
1.1	0	0	0	0	97	97	97	37	24	16
1.0	0	10	3	49	91	96	98	78	82	72
0.9	0	1	15	81	97	97	**96**	96	72	83
0.8	0	16	15	79	96	97	90	92	70	37
0.6	0	10	24	71	74	48	29	79	61	14
0.4	0	7	26	41	45	42	40	80	14	26
0.2	0	3	14	29	39	33	20	26	24	14
0	0	5	13	14	24	24	52	27	62	14

Glycerol (v/v %)

90% Recovery for HUGGINS-Frozen Red Cells

2) Glyceool-Rapid

NaCl (w/v %)

NaCl	0	10	20	30	40	50	60	70	80	90
18.0	0	14	0	15	10	8	12	0	1	92
12.0	0	2	8	2	14	50	70	60	82	91
9.0	0	0	0	0	17	84	83	90	66	92
7.0	0	7	12	72	90	94	83	75	90	90
5.0	0	15	50	51	96	95	87	95	92	73
4.0	0	5	7	38	91	96	91	92	92	66
3.6	0	5	6	65	97	90	90	90	89	63
3.2	0	0	14	35	96	97	95	91	85	90
3.8	0	1	15	72	95	96	93	90	93	87
2.4	0	0	26	95	96	95	94	94	93	59
2.0	0	68	83	94	93	94	93	90	36	27
1.8	0	23	97	95	94	66	72	26	12	4
1.6	0	24	51	97	96	80	64	23	22	19
1.4	0	37	94	93	90	93	91	21	5	5
1.2	0	64	90	93	76	85	89	13	0	4
1.0	0	15	88	90	66	84	86	12	0	5
0.8	0	20	91	83	73	83	57	5	0	1
0.6	0	56	86	51	71	50	49	0	9	16
0.4	0	32	70	46	33	17	19	1	0	3
0.2	0	4	0	0	0	0	2	0	0	0
0	0	0	0	0	1	0	0	0	0	0

Glycerol (v/v %)

97% Recovery for ROWE-Frozen Red Cells

3) DMSO-Slow

NaCl (w/v %)

NaCl	10	20	40	50	60	70	80	90
9.0	20	35	21	46	47	55	35	20
5.0	6	17	45	63	86	92	32	35
4.0	0	0	35	50	88	79	23	15
3.2	0	0	0	27	80	88	0	0
2.8	0	0	0	56	85	64	29	1
2.4	0	0	40	9	91	33	15	0
2.0	0	0	0	48	88	43	27	0
1.8	0	0	9	83	84	49	3	0
1.6	0	0	75	88	64	29	7	0
1.4	0	0	65	92	84	65	0	0
1.2	0	0	67	93	93	83	5	0
1.0	0	0	49	95	94	86	19	13
0,8	0	5	85	87	74	39	7	0
0.6	10	26	31	42	13	16	9	0
0.4	6	21	25	41	56	16	7	5
0.2	0	0	0	0	0	5	1	1

DMSO (v/v %)

94% Recovery for HUGGINS-Frozen Red Cells

4) DMSO-Rapid

NaCl (w/v %)

NaCl	10	20	30	40	50	60	70	80	90
18.0	4	15	29	49	46	43	42	40	23
9.0	0	16	20	45	68	70	41	62	41
5.0	0	23	81	88	93	94	82	82	20
4.0	0	42	74	94	95	93	79	87	33
3.2	0	6	81	92	96	89	87	67	16
2.8	0	47	84	93	96	89	84	40	4
2.4	0	47	87	90	94	89	76	73	0
2.0	0	46	91	92	91	88	87	73	21
1.8	0	84	93	95	96	89	92	78	27
1.6	0	90	96	97	95	91	88	83	15
1.4	6	88	95	95	95	91	88	57	21
1.2	16	95	97	96	94	88	80	46	22
1.0	13	95	95	96	90	90	73	61	8
0.8	30	95	96	93	92	85	43	37	24
0.6	35	95	95	86	86	60	30	30	26
0.4	34	90	85	53	45	26	30	31	28
0.2	29	39	18	18	21	18	15	22	13

DMSO (v/v %)

97% Recovery for ROWE-Frozen Red Cells

Fig. 58 Recovery of rapidly and slowly cooled red blood cells. Cryoprotectant was dissolved in the salt solution in water (w/v %) to make the respective concentrations (w/v %) of cryoprotective solution. Each cryoprotective solution was added to the same volume of packed red cells in a limited 5 minutes. For the slow-freezing, the glycerolized red cells in a 120 mm polyethylene tube, outer diameter 12 mm, wall thickness 1 mm were cooled by 0.3–0.4 C per

5) Ethylene glycol-Slow

NaCl (w/v %)

	10	20	40	50	60	70	80	90
3.2	0	0	0	16	22	76	85	22
2.8	0	0	0	0	45	86	88	18
2.4	0	0	0	39	51	87	82	7
2.0	0	4	0	36	72	87	55	0
1.8	0	0	0	67	84	90	61	0
1.6	0	0	12	60	92	91	73	0
1.4	0	0	20	74	91	89	20	0
1.2	0	0	50	89	94	81	11	0
1.0	0	0	31	85	91	64	0	0
0.8	0	0	58	89	73	3	0	0
0.6	0	0	59	55	24	9	0	0
0.4	0	0	48	19	6	0	0	0
0.2	0	3	5	0	0	0	0	0
0	0	0	0	0	0	0	0	0

Ethylene glycol (v/v %)

93% Recovery for HUGGINS-Frozen Red Cells

6) Ethylene glycol-Rapid

NaCl (w/v %)

	10	20	30	40	50	60	70	80	90
3.2	5	70	8	67	46	4	7	1	14
2.8	13	17	79	20	8	52	63	20	30
2.4	1	25	71	52	27	55	28	26	6
2.0	0	49	2	4	75	18	52	17	16
1.8	4	68	9	20	70	25	11	24	11
1.6	2	76	10	24	59	11	16	40	42
1.4	0	19	63	43	17	66	46	43	37
1.2	0	59	4	56	9	0	0	0	0
1.0	5	4	17	67	36	4	0	0	9
0.8	9	58	40	33	8	0	9	4	1
0.6	13	12	13	23	9	11	4	7	11
0.4	9	5	25	2	0	5	8	1	0
0.2	0	4	4	0	0	0	0	0	0

Ethylene glycol (v/v %)

94% Recovery for ROWE-Frozen Red Cells

7) Sucrose-Slow

NaCl (w/v %)

	10	20	40	50	60	70	80	90
3.2	0	3	11	16	13	17	2	1
2.8	0	3	0	6	7	5	3	1
2.4	0	0	5	0	12	17	27	8
2.0	0	0	0	2	4	0	25	25
1.8	0	1	0	0	0	9	20	9
1.6	0	0	0	0	3	1	5	13
1.4	0	0	0	0	0	17	19	15
1.2	0	0	0	0	0	6	16	1
1.0	0	0	0	1	0	1	0	0
0.8	0	0	0	0	3	16	1	0
0.6	0	0	0	0	5	16	8	6
0.4	0	0	0	0	0	11	9	0
0.2	0	0	0	2	0	15	5	1
0.1	0	0	0	0	0	6	1	0

Sucrose (v/v %)

97% Recovery for HUGGINS-Frozen Red Cells

8) Sucrose-Rapid

NaCl (w/v) %

	10	20	30	40	50	60	70	80	90
3.2	2	9	16	15	16	37	31	23	16
2.8	0	5	7	5	5	40	42	38	23
2.4	0	13	13	9	16	31	26	31	2
2.0	0	0	0	0	16	0	28	12	5
1.8	0	5	0	2	12	6	16	5	0
1.6	0	0	5	0	5	17	9	14	0
1.4	0	7	9	2	8	7	19	14	0
1.2	0	3	14	6	0	12	5	0	0
1.0	0	0	3	2	0	8	0	5	0
0.8	0	16	6	3	5	4	20	11	1
0.6	1	0	13	7	5	23	26	13	0
0.4	0	0	9	0	0	17	12	9	0
0.2	0	2	9	0	4	19	9	3	0
0.1	0	0	0	0	0	8	1	0	0

Sucrose (v/v %)

95% Recovery for ROWE-Frozen Red Cells

minute to $-80°C$ by use of a fully automated device for temperature controlled freezing. For the rapid-freezing, the glycerolized red cells were directly transferred into liquid nitrogen manually, and cooled by $200°C$ per minute to $-196°C$. Thawing was accomplished in a water bath at $+40°C$ within 2 minutes, HUGGINS' and ROWE's solution were used respectively as the controls. Recovery rate was calculated by the following formula:

$$\% \text{ recovery} = \frac{\text{Supernatant hemoglobin concentration after thawing}}{\text{Total content of hemoglobin before freezing}} \times 200$$

For example, the 60% glycerol in 0.9% salt solution produced a 96% recovery by the slow-freezing, and the 30% glycerol in 1.0% salt solutio a 90% recovery by the rapid-freezing. Ninety percent recoveries are framed. These figures show that glycerol has a wide area of 90% and over recovery wherever slowly or rapidly cooled. DMSO, however, has the narrower area of the 90% recovery in the show freezing, Ethylene glycol has remarkably narrow area of the 90% recovery. Sucrose does not produce the 90% recovery.

References

BALDINI, M. G.: Discussion on the current status of platelet preservation. *Cryobiology*, **5**: 49–57, 1968.

BEUTLER, E. and WOOD, L.: The *in vivo* regeneration of red cell 2, 3-diphosphoglyceric acid (DPG) after transfusion of stored blood. *J. Laborat. Clin. Med.*, **74**: 300–304, 1969.

BRICKA, M. and BESSIS, M.: Sur la conservation des érythrocytes par congélation à basse température en présence de polyvinylpyrrolidone et de dextran. *Comp. Rend. Soc. Biol.* (Paris), **149**: 875–877, 1955.

BOWMAN, S.: Red cell preservation in citrate-phosphate-dextrose and in acid-citrate-dextrose: comparison of erythrocyte viability after 28 days refrigerated storage. *Transfusion*, **3**: 364–367, 1963.

BRIKHOUS, K. M., SHERMER, R. W. and MOSTOFI, F. K. (eds.): The platelets (International Academy of Pathology, Monograph No. 11), The Williams & Wilkins Co., Baltimore, 1971.

CALLOWAY, N. O. and MOWREY, F. H.: Red blood cells as course of protein for parenteral use. *J. Amer. Med. Ass.*, **152**: 777–781, 1953.

CHAPLIN, H., JR. and VEALL, N.: Removal of glycerol from previously frozen red cells. *Lancet*, I: 218–219, 1953a.

CHAPLIN, H., JR. and MOLLISON, P. L.: Improved storage of red cells at −20°C. *Lancet*, I: 215–216, 1953b.

CHAPLAIN, H., JR., CRAWFORD, H., CUBUSH, M. and MOLLISON, P. L.: Post-transfusion survival of red cells stored at −20°C. *Lancet*, I: 852–858, 1954.

CHAPLIN, H., JR., CRAWFORD, H., CUTBUSH, M. and MOLLISON, P. L.: Preservation of red cell at −79°C. *Clin. Sci.*, **15**: 27–39, 1956.

CHAPLIN, H., JR., SCHMIDT, P. J. and STEINFELD, J. L.: Storage of red cells at sub-zero temperatures, Further studies. *Clin. Sci.*, **16**: 651–661, 1957.

COHEN, P. and GARDNER, F. H.: Canine platelet lifespan after freezing with glycerin-plasma solution. *J. Clin. Invest.*, **38**: 995–996, 1959 (Abstract).

COHEN, P. and GARDNER, F. H.: Platelet preservation. I. Preservation of canine platelets at 4°C. *J. Clin. Invest.*, **41**: 1–9, 1962.

COHEN, P. and GARDNER, F. H.: Platelet preservation of canine platelet concentrates by freezing in solution of glycerol-plasma. *J. Clin. Invest.*, **41**: 10–19, 1962.

COHEN, P. and GARDNER, F. H.: Platelet preservation. IV. Preservation of human platelet concentrates by controlled slow freezing in a glycerol medium. *New England J. Med,.* **274**: 1400–1407, 1966.

CRAWFORD, H. and MOLLISON, P. L.: Reversal of electrolyte changes in stored red cells after transfusion. *J. Physiol.* (London), **129**: 639–647, 1955.

DACIE, J. V. and MOLLISON, P. L.: Survival of normal erythrocytes after transfusion to patients with familiar haemolytic anaemia (acholuric jaundice), *Lancet*, I: 550–552, 1943.

DANNE, T. A., VALERI, C. R. and BARTON, R. K.: Autotransfusion of previously frozen blood in elective gynecologic surgery. *Amer. J. Obstet. Gynecol.*, **105**: 394–399, 1969.

DERRICK, J. B., LIND, M. and ROWE, A. W.: Studies of the metabolic integrity of human red blood cells after cryopreservation. I. Effects of low-glycerol-rapid-freeze preservation on energy status and intracellular sodium and potassium. *Transfusion*, **9**: 317–323, 1969.

DILLER, K. R. and CRAVALHO, E. G.: A cryomicroscope for the freezing and thawing processes in biological cells. *Cryobiology*, **7**: 191–199, 1970.

DJERASSI, I. and ROY, A.: Preservation of viable platelets in the frozen state. *Life Sci.*, **1**: 237–331, 1962.

DJERASSI, I. and ROY, A.:   A method for preservation of viable platelets: combined effects of sugars and dimethylsulfoxide. *Blood,* **22**: 703–717, 1962.

DJERASSI, I., ROY, A. and ALVARADO, J.:   Preservation of morphological integrity and clot retraction activity of human platelets after freezing. *Thromb. Diath. Haemorrh.,* **11**: 222–229, 1964.

DJERASSI, I., FARBER, S., ROY, A. and CAVINS, J.:   Preparation and *in vivo* circulation of human platelets preserved with combined dimethylsulfoxide and dextrose. *Transfusion,* **6**: 572–576, 1966.

DJERASSI, I., ROY, A., KIM, J. and CAVINS, J.:   Dimethylacetamide, a new cryophylactic agent for platelets. *Transfusion,* **11**: 72–76, 1871.

DOEBBLER, G. F. and RINFRET, A. P.:   The influence of protective compounds and cooling and warming conditions on hemolysis of erythrocytes by freezing and thawing. *Biochim. Biophys. Acta,* **58**: 449–458, 1962.

DOEBBLER, G. F.:   Symposium on cryoprotective agents. *Cryobiology,* **3**: 1, 1966a.

DOEBBLER, G. F.:   Cryoprotective compounds. Review and discussion of structure and function. *Cryobiology,* **3**: 2–11, 1966b.

FARRANT, J.:   Mechanism of cell damage during freezing and thawing and its preservation. *Nature* (London), **205**: 1284–1287, 1965.

FIRKIN, B. G., ARIMURA, G. and HARRINGTON, W. J.:   A method for evaluating the hemostatic effect of various agent in thrombocytopenic rat and mice. *Blood,* **15**: 388–394, 1960.

FLIEDNER, T. M., SORENSON, D. K., BOND, V. P., CRONKITE, E. P., JACKSON, D. P. and ADAMIK, E.:   Comparative effectiveness of fresh and lyophilized platelets in controlling irradiation hemorrhage in rat. *Proc. Soc. Exper. Biol. Med.,* **99**: 731–733, 1958.

FLORIO, L., STEWART, M. and MUGRAGE, E. R.:   The effect of freezing on erythrocytes. *J. Laborat. Clin. Med.,* **28**: 1486–1490, 1942.

GABRIO, B. W., HENNESSEY, M., THOMASSON, J. and FINCH, C. A.:   Erythrocyte preservation. IV. *In vitro* reversibility of the storage lession. *J. Biol. Chem.,* **215**: 357–367, 1955.

GABRIO, B. W., DONOHUE, D. M., HUENNEKENS, F. M. and FINCH, C. A.:   Erythrocytes preservation. VII. Acid-Citrate-Dextrose-Inosine (ACDI) as a preservative for blood during storage at 4°C. *J. Clin. Invest.,* **35**: 657–663, 1956.

GARDNER, F. H.:   Platelet preservation problems. *Cryobiology,* **5**: 42–48, 1968.

GIBSON, J. G.:   Blood component therapy. The bulletin of the South Central Association of Blood Banks. December 3–12, 1959.

GREIFF, D. and MACKEY, S.:   Cryobiology of platelets. II. The effects of freezing and storage at low temperatures on the survival of isolated human blood platelets as measured by assays for aminopeptidases. *Cryobiology,* **7**: 9–13, 1970.

HENDERSON, I. W. D.:   Cold injury and oxdative phosphorylation. The 7th Annual Meeting of the Society for Cryobiology (Abstract), **6**(6):581–582, 1970.

HENNESSEY, M., FINCH, C. A. and GABRIO, B. W.:   Erythrocyte preservation. VIII. Metabolic degradation of nucleosides *in vitro* and *in vivo*. *J. Clin. Invest.,* **36**: 429–433, 1957.

HUGGINS, C. E.:   Reversible agglomeration used to remove dimethylsulfoxide from large volumes of frozen blood. *Science,* **139**: 504–505, 1963.

HUGGINS, C. E.:   Frozen blood. *Ann. Surg.,* **160**: 643–649, 1964.

HUGGINS, C. E. and GROVE-RUSMSSEN, M.:   Advances in blood preservation. *Postgrad. Med.,* **37**: 557–569, 1965.

HUGGINS, C. E.:   Frozen blood. *J. Japan. Soc. Blood Transfusion,* **12**: 67–78, 1965.

HUGGINS, C. E.:   Frozen blood—clinical experience. *Surgery,* **60**: 77–84, 1966.

HUGGINS, C. E.:   Preservation of storage of blood. In: Human transplantation, ed. by RAPAPORT, F. T. and DAUSSET, J., pp. 669–674, Grune & Stratton, New York and London, 1968.

HUGGINS, C. E.:   Frozen blood. *Europ. Surg. Res.,* **1**: 3, 1969, cited from S. G. O. October: 910, 1969.

IOSSIFIDES, I. A., GEISLER, P., EICHMAN, M. F. and TOCANTINS, L. M.:   Preservation of platelets with demethylsulfoxide in the frozen state. *Blood,* **20**: 762–763, 1962 (Abstract).

JACKSON, D. P., SORENSON, D. K., CRONKITE, E. P., BOND, V. P. and FLIEDNER, T. M.: Effectiveness of transfusion of fresh and lyophilized platelets in controlling bleeding due to thrombocytepenia. *J. Clin. Invest.*, **38**: 1689–1697, 1959.

JONES, N. C. H., MOLLISON, P. L. and ROBINSON, M. A.: Factors affecting the viability of erythrocytes stored in the frozen state. *Proc. Roy. Soc. Biol. Sci.*, **147**: 476–497, 1957.

KAROW, A. M.: Cryoprotectants. A new class of drugs. *J. Pharmacy. Pharmacol.*, **21**: 209–223, 1969.

KETCHEL, M. M., TULLIS, J. L., TINCH, R. J., DRISCOLL, S. G. and SNEGENOR, D. M.: Use of biomechanical equipment for the long-term preservation of erythrocytes. *J. Amer. Med. Ass.*, **168**: 404–498, 1958.

KLEIN, E., TOCH, R., FARBER, S., FREEMAN, G. and FIORENTINO, R.: Hemostasis in thrombocytopenic bleeding following infusion of stored, frozen platelets. *Blood*, **11**: 693–699, 1956a.

KLEIN, E., FARBER, S., DJERASSI, I., TOCH, R., FREEMAN, G. and ARNOLD, P.: The preparation and clinical administration of lyophilized platelet material to children with acute leucemia and aplastic anemia. *J. Pediatrics*, **49**: 517–522, 1956b.

KLIMAN, A.: No hepatitis after red cells? *New England J. Med.*, **279**: 1290, 1968.

KO, I.: Studies on electronmicroscopic findings (low power) of frozen red cells. *J. Japan. Soc. Blood Transfusion*, **16**(6): 215–229, 1969 (in Japanese with English summary).

KÖRNER, W. F., KLEINE, N.: Der Einfluß von Vitamin E auf die Stabilität der Erythrozyten und die praktische Anwendung dieser Erkenntnis für die Blutkonservierung. *Int. Zeitschrt. Vitaminforsch.*, **35**: 138–152, 1965.

KOWALSKI, E. and NIEWIAROWSKI, S.: Biochemistry of blood platelets. Academic Press, London and New York, 1967.

KREVANS, J. R.: Survival of platelets transfused into thrombocytopenic recipients. In: Blood platelets, ed. by JOHNSON, S. A., MONTO, R. W., REBUCK, J. W. and HORN, R. C., JR., pp. 651–655, Little Brown and Company, Boston, 1961.

KRIJNEN, H. W., DE WIT, J. J. FR. M., KUIVENHOVEN, A. C. J. and REYDEN, G. V. D.: Freezing of red cells with liquid nitrogen. I. Result with glycerol as an intracellular substance. Proceedings of the 10th Congress International Society on Blood Transfusion, Stockholm (1964), pp. 683–686, 1965.

KRIJNEN, H. W. KUIVENHOVEN, A. C. J. and DE WIT, J. J. FR. M.: The preservation of blood cells in the frozen state. Experiences and current methods in the Netherlands. *Cryobiology*, **5**: 136–143, 1968.

KRIJNEN, H. W., GONDSMIT, R., DE WIT, J. J. FR. M., KUIVENHOVEN, A. C. J. and PRINS, H. K.: Some experiences with the preservation of frozen glycerolized red cells. Proceedings of the 11th Congress International Society on Blood Transfusion, Sydney (1966): *Bibl. Haemat.* No. 29, Part 3, pp. 807–813, (Karger, Basel/New York, 1968).

KUROKAWA, I., KIMURA, T., YAMAMOTO, E., SATO, N. and NAGAI, T.: Studies on the effect of Vitamin E upon the preservation of blood. I. Vitamin (Japan) **38**: 10–11, 1968, II. Vitamins (Japan) **39**: 11–13, 1969, III. Vitamins (Japan) **39**: 86–90, 1969, IV. Vitamins (Japan) **40**: 202–205, 1969, V. Vitamins (Japan) **40**: 206–209, 1969 (in Japanese with English summary).

LOVELOCK, J. E.: The haemolysis of human red blood cells by freezing and thawing. *Biochim. Biophys. Acta*, **10**: 414–426, 1953a.

LOVELOCK, J. E.: The mechanism of the protective action of glycerol against haemolysis by freezing and thawing. *Biochim. Biophys. Acta*, **11**: 28–36, 1953b.

LOVELOCK, J. E.: Physical instability and thermal shock in red cells. *Nature* (London), **173**: 659–661, 1954a.

LOVELOCK, J. E.: The protective action of neutral solutes against haemolysis by freezing and thawing. *Biochem. J.*, **56**: 265–270, 1954b.

LOVELOCK, J. E. and POLGE, C.: The immobilization of spermatozoa by freezing and thawing and the protective action of glycerol. *Biochem. J.*, **58**: 618–622, 1954c.

LOVELOCK, J. E.: Haemolysis by thermal shock. *Brit. J. Haemat.*, **1**: 117–129, 1955a.

LOVELOCK, J. E.: The physical instability of human red blood cells. *Biochem. J.*, **60**: 692–696, 1955b.

LOVELOCK, J. E.: The physical instability of human red blood cells and its possiple importance in their senescence. Ciba Foundation Colloq. on Ageing, **2**: 215–232, 1956.

LOVELOCK, J. E.: Denaturation of lipid-protein complexes as a cause of damage py freezing. *Proc. Roy. Soc. Biol. Sci.*, **147**: 427–433, 1957.

LOVELOCK, J. E. and BISHOP, M. W. H.: Prevention of freezing damage to living cells by dimethylsulfoxide. *Nature* (London), **183**: 1394–1395, 1959.

LUNDBERG, A., PERT, J. and ZUCKER, M.: *In vitro* testings of frozen blood platelets. American Association of Blood Banks 19th Annual Meeting, Los Angeles, 1968.

LUYET, B. J. and HODAPP, E. L.: Revival of frog's spermatozoa vitrified in liquid air. *Proc. Soc. Exper. Biol. Med.*, **39**: 433–435, 1938.

LUYET, B. J. and HARTUNG, M. C.: Factors in the revival of anguillula aceti after its solidification in liquid air. *Amer. J. Physiol.*, **133**: 368–369, 1941.

LUYET, B. J.: Ultra-rapid freezing as a possible method of blood preservation. In: Preservation of the formed elements and of the proteins of the blood, pp. 141–146, American Red Cross, Washington, D. C., 1959.

LUYET, B. J. and PRIBOR, D.: Direct observation of hemolysis during the rewarming and thawing of frozen blood. *Biodynamica*, **196**: 319–332, 1965.

LUYET, B. J.: Attacks from different fronts on some complex cases of inectability in aqueous solutions solidified at low temperatures. Physics of snow and ice. Proceedings of the International Conference on Low Temperature Science, ed. by OURA, H., Vol. 1, Part 1, The Institute of Low Temperature Science, Hokkaido University, Sapporo, 1966a.

LUYET, B. J.: Various modes of recrystallization of ice. Physics of snow and ice. Proceedings of the International Conference on Low Temperature Science, ed. by OURA, H., Vol. 1, Part 1. The Institute of Low Temperature Science, Hokkaido University, Sapporo, 1966b.

LUYET, B. J.: Preservation and storage of living cells at low temperatures. In: Human transplantation, ed. by RAPAPORT, F. T. and DAUSSET, J., pp. 655–668, Grune & Stratton, New York and London, 1968.

MARCUS, A. J. and ZUCKER, M. B.: The physiology of blood platelets. Grune & Stratton, New York and London, 1965.

MATSUBARA, T., OKUZONO, H. and TAMAGAWA, S.: Proposal for an improved reagent in the hemoglobin cyanide method. The 13th International Congress of Hematology, August 2–8, 1970, Munich.

MATSUDA, T., TAUBE, R. R., DERN, R. J., et al.: Red cell survival of 42 day acid-citrate-dextrose (ACD) -adenine preserved blood after transfusion into traumatized patients. *J. Laborat. Clin. Med.*, **72**: 42–46, 1969.

MERYMAN, H. T. and KAFIG, E.: Rapid freezing and thawing of whole blood. *Proc. Soc. Exper. Biol. Med.*, **90**: 587–589, 1955.

MERYMAN, H. T.: Preservation of blood by freezing. A review. *Cryobiology*, **1**: 52–56, 1964.

MERYMAN, H. T. (ed.): Cryobiology. Academic Press, London and New York, 1966.

MERYMAN, H. T.: Observations on the present state of blood preservation by freezing. *Cryobiology*, **5**: 144–146, 1968.

MERYMAN, H. T.: Absence of unfrozen freezable water in rapidly frozen red cells. *Cryobiology*, **7**: 252–255, 1970.

MERYMAN, H. T.: Cryoprotective agents. *Cryobiology*, **8** 173–183, 1971.

MINAKAMI, S., OHYAMA, H. and YOSHIKAWA, H.: Changes of glycolytic intermediates of erythrocytes during storage in acid citrate dextrose medium. *Folia Haemat.*, **91**: 115–123, 1969.

MIURA, T.: A new type of cytoaglomerator for frozen blood processing. *J. Japan. Med. Instrument*, **37**: 489, 1967a (in Japanese).

MIURA, T.: Frozen blood. *J. Japan. Soc. Blood transfusion*, **16**: 185–191, 1969b (in Japanese).

MIURA, T., NINOMIYA, K., MIZUNO, A. and HATANO, S.: Clinical application of frozen blood. The 12th International Congress on Blood Transfusion, Abstract, August 17–23, 1969 (Moscow). "MIR" Publ., Moscow, 1969c.

MOLLISON, P. L. and SLOVITER, H. A.: Successful transfusion of previously frozen human red cells. *Lancet,* **II**: 862–864, 1951.

MOLLISON, P. L., SLOVITER, H. A. and CHAPLIN, H., JR.: Survival of transfused red cells previously stored for long periods in the frozen state. *Lancet,* **II**: 501–505, 1952.

MOLLISON, P. L. and VEALL, N.: The use of the isotope ^{51}Cr as a label for red cells. *Brit. J. Haemat.,* **1**: 62–74, 1955.

MORRISON, F. S.: Preservation of blood platelets current methods. *Cryobiology,* **5**: 29–41, 1968.

MOSKOWITZ, M. and CALVIN, M.: On the components and structure of the human red cell membrane. *Exper. Cell Res.,* **3**: 33–46, 1952.

MOSS, G. S., VALERI, C. R. and BRODINE, C. E.: Clinical experience with the use of frozen blood in combat causalties. *New England J. Med.,* **278**: 747–752, 1968.

MOSS, G. S.: Massive transfusion of frozen processed red cells in combat causalties. Reports of three cases. *Surgery,* **66**: 1008–1013, 1969.

MURRAY, C. K., HALE, D. E. and SHAAR, C. M.: The preparation and use of red blood cell suspensions in treatment of anemia. *J. Amer. Med. Ass.,* **122**: 1065–1067, 1943.

NAKAO, M., NAKAO, T., TATIBANA, M., YOSHIKAWA, H. and ABE, T.: Effect of inosine and adenin on adenosine triphosphate regeneration and shape transformation in long-stored erythrocytes. *Biochim. Biophys. Acta,* **32**: 564–565, 1959.

NAKAO, M. and NAKAO, T.: A new preservative medium maintaining the level of adenosine triphosphate and the osmotic resistance erythrocyte. *Proc. Japan. Acad.,* **36**: 43–47, 1960.

NEI, T.: Mechanism of hemolysis of erythrocytes by freezing at near-zero temperature. I. Microscopic observation of hemolyzing erythrocytes during the freezing and thawing process. *Cryobiology,* **4**: 153–156, 1967.

NEI, T.: Mechanism of hemolysis of erythrocytes by freezing, with special reference to freezing at near-zero temperature. In: The frozen cell, A Ciba Foundation Symposium on the Frozen Cell, ed. by WOLSTENHOLME, G. E. W. and O'CONNOR, H., J. & A. Churchill, London, 1970.

PERRAULT, R., JACKSON, J. R., MARTIN-VILLAR, J. and SMILEY, R. K.: Experience with the use of frozen blood. *Canad. Med. Ass. J.,* **96**: 1504–1509, 1967.

PERT, J. H., SCHORK, P. K. and MOORE, R.: A new method of low-temperature blood preservation using liquid nitrogen and a glycerol-sucrose additive. *Clin. Res.,* **11**: 197, 1963 (Abstract).

PFISTERER, H., WEBER, F. and MICHLMAYR, G.: *In vivo* survival of platelet concentrates following rapid freezing and thawing. *Cryobiology.* **5**: 379–384, 1969.

POLGE, C., SMITH, A. U. and PARKES, A. S.: Revival of spermatozoa after vitrification and dehydration at low temperatures. *Nature* (London), **164**: 666, 1949.

PYLE, H. M.: Glycerol preservation of red cells. *Cryobiology,* **1**: 57–60, 1964.

RACCUGLIA, G. and BETHELL, F. H.: Platelet transfusion and administration of platelet derivatives in man. II. Evaluation of systemic hemostatic properties of various preparations. *Amer. J. Clin. Path.,* **34**: 505–512, 1960.

RACCUGLIN, G. and ZARAFONETIS, C. J. D.: Pharmacologic compounds, fresh and preserved platelets in experimental thrombocytopenia. In: Proceedings of the 9th Congress International Society on Blood Transfusion, pp. 34–41, Mexico City, 1962.

RAPATZ, G. and LUYET, B.: Combined effects of freezing rates and of various protective agents on the preservation of human erythrocytes. *Cryobiology,* **4**: 215–222, 1968.

REBUCK, J. W.: Blood platelets. *Transfusion,* **3**: 1–5, 1963.

RINFRET, A. P.: Factors affecting the erythrocyte during rapid freezing and thawing. *Ann. N. Y. Acad. Sci.,* **85**: 576–594, 1960.

ROWE, A. W., EYSTER, E. and KELLNER, A.: Liquid nitrogen preservation of red blood cells for transfusion. *Cryobiology,* **5**: 119–128, 1968.

ROWE, A. W., DERRICK, J. B., MILES, W., ALLEN, F. H., JR. and KELLNER, A.: The biochemistry and clinical use of red cells frozen by the low glycerol-rapid freeze technique, modern problems of blood preservation. Proceedings of International Symposium of Modern Problems of Blood Transfusion, held at the Department of Immunohaematology and Blood

Transfusion, Jahann Wolfgang Goethe University Frankfurt/Main (1968), March 17th–18th, pp. 184–198, Gustav Fischer Verlag, Stuttgart, 1969.

SLOVITER, H. A.: Recovery of human red-blood-cells after freezing. *Lancet*, I: 823–824, 1951.

SLOVITER, H. A.: *In vivo* survival of rabbit's red cells recovered after freezing. *Lancet*, I: 1350–1351, 1951.

SLOVITER, H. A.: Recovery of human red cells after prolonged storage at −79°C. *Nature* (London), **169**: 1013–1014, 1952.

SLOVITER, H. A.: A method for preparing thawed erythrocyte-glycerol mixtures for transfusion. *Amer. J. Med. Sci.*, **231**: 437–440, 1956.

SLOVITER, H. A.: Effects of the intravenous administration of glycerol solutions to animals and man. *J. Clin. Invest.*, **37**: 619–626, 1958.

SLOVITER, H. A.: The transfusion of erythrocyte-glycerol mixtures after prolonged storage at low temperatures. Proceedings of the 15th Congress on Military Medicine, Beograd, pp. 429–432, 1959.

SMITH, A. U.: Prevention of hemolysis during freezing and thawing of red blood cells. *Lancet*, II: 901–911, 1950.

SMITH, A. U., POLGE, C. and SMILES, J.: Microscopic observation of living cells during freezing and thawing. *J. Roy. Microsc. Soc.*, **71**: 186–195, 1951.

SMITH, A. U. and SMILES, J.: Microscopic studies of mammalian tissues during cooling to −79°C. *J. Roy. Microsc. Soc.*, **73**: 134–139, 1953.

SMITH, A. U.: Effects of low temperature on living cells and tissues. In: Biological Applications of Freezing and Drying, Chap. I, ed. by HARRIS, R. J. C., Academic Press, London and New York, 1954.

SMITH, A. U.: Biological effects of freezing and supercooling, Edward Arnold Publ., London, 1961.

STEWART, G. J. and TURNER, H. M.: Ultrastructural characteristics and behavior of previously frozen, glycerolized and deglycerolized human red blood cells. *Cryobiology*, **4**: 189–196, 1968.

STRUMIA, M. M. (ed.): General principles of blood transfusion. *Transfusion*, **3**: 303–346, 1963.

STRUMIA, M. M.: Preservation of red cells in the frozen state with sugars and macromolecular additives. Progress report No. 58. Mechanism of injury of freezing. John S. Sharpe Research Foundation, Bryn Mawr Hospital, Bryn Mawr, Pa., 1965.

STRUMIA, M. M.: Preservation of red cells in the frozen state with sugars and macromolecular additives. Progress report No. 60. Effects of physical factors on red cells subject to freezing and thawing. John S. Sharpe Research Foundation, Bryn Mawr Hospital, Bryn Mawr, Pa., 1966.

STRUMIA, M. M.: Platelet preservation. *Cryobiology*, **5**: 58–59, 1968.

SUMIDA, S.: Frozen blood and serum hepatitis, *Igaku-no-ayumi*, **57**: 757–758, 1966 (in Japanese).

SUMIDA, S. and OKUYAMA, Y.: Serum hepatitis from frozen blood transfusion. *Igaku-no-ayumi*, **63**: 245–246, 1967 (in Japanese).

SUMIDA, S., OKUYAMA, Y. and KAMEGAI, T.: Serum hepatitis from frozen blood. *Lancet*, II: 1255–1256, 1967.

SUMIDA, S.: Frozen blood processing apparatus. *J. Japan. Med. Instrument*, **37**: 458–488, 1967 (in Japanese).

SUMIDA, S., KO, I., SHIBANO, R., KASHIWADA, K., TASHIRO, M. and OKUYAMA, Y.: Studies on freeze-preservation of erythrocytes. *J. Japan. Soc. Blood Transfusion*, **14**: 231–233, 1967 (in Japanese).

SUMIDA, S.: Hemoglobinuria from frozen blood. *Igaku-no-ayumi*, **67**: 587–588, 1968 (in Japanese).

SUMIDA, S.: A standard method of frozen blood transfusion. *J. Japan. Accident Med. Ass.*, **17**: 46–54, 1969 (in Japanese).

SUMIDA, S.: The freshness of red cells to be frozen and the deglycerolization. *Japan. Soc. for Research of Freezing and Drying*, **15**: 10–16, 1969 (in Japanese).

SUMIDA, S.: Studies on the rapid-freeze procedure of red cells. *Japan. Soc. for Research of Freezing and Drying*, **16**: 42–46, 1970 (in Japanese).

SUMIDA, S.: A new equipment for frozen blood processing. *J. Japan. Med. Instrument*, **40**(7): 542–545, 1970 (in Japanese).

SUMIDA, S.: Clinical experiences of frozen platelet transfusion. *Igaku-no-ayumi*, **75**(1): 18–19, 1970 (in Japanese).

SUMIDA, S. and YOSHINARI, M.: Side effects of frozen blood transfusion. *Nippon Iji-shinpo*, **2478**: 26–32, 1971 (in Japanese).

SUMIDA, S.: Frozen blood (Movie film, 16 mm, optical sound, color, 15 minutes long), 1969.

SUMIDA, S.: Frozen blood (Movie film, 16 mm, optical sound, color, 18 minutes long), 1970.

SUMIDA, S.: Frozen blood component therapy (Movie film, 16 mm, optical sound, color, 19 minutes long), 1971.

SZYMANSKI, I. O. and VALERI, C. R.: Automated differential agglutination technic to measure red cell survival. II. Survival *in vivo* of preserved red cells. *Transfusion*, **8**(2): 74–83, 1968.

TATIBANA, M., SHIMANUNE, A. NAKAO, M., ISHII, Y., HASHIMOTO, T. and YOSHIKAWA, H.: Potassium uptake and glycolytic activity of human erythrocytes with various adenosinetriphosphate concentrations. *Folia Haemat.*, **79**: 470–474, 1962.

TULLIS, J. L.: Preservation of platelets. *Amer. J. Med. Sci.*, **226**: 191–202, 1953.

TULLIS, J. L., KETCHEL, M. M., PYLE, H. M., PENNEL, R. B., GIBSON, J. G., II, TINCH, R. J. and DRISCOLL, S. G.: Studies on the *in vivo* survival of glycerolized and frozen human red blood cells. *J. Amer. Med. Ass.*, **168**: 399–404, 1958.

TULLIS, J. L., SURGENOR, D. M. and BAUDANZA, P.: Preserved platelets: their preparation, storage and clinical use. *Blood*, **14**: 456–475, 1959.

TULLIS, J. L. and LIONETTI, F. J.: Preservation of blood by freezing. *Anesthesiology*, **27**: 483–493, 1966.

TULLIS, J. L., HINMAN, J., SPROUL, M. T. and NICKERSON, R. J.: Incidence of posttransfusion hepatitis in previously frozen blood. *J. Amer. Med. Ass.*, **214**: 719–723, 1970.

TURNER, A. R.: Frozen blood, Gordon & Breach, New York and London, 1970.

VALERI, C. R., RUNCK, A. H. and SAMPSON, W. T.: Effects of agglomeration human red blood cells. *Transfusion*, **9**: 120–134, 1969.

VALERI, C. R.: Frozen blood. *New England J. Med.*, **275**: 365–431, 1966.

VALERI, C. R.: Frozen blood (Concluded). *New England J. Med.*, **275**: 425–431, 1966.

VALERI, C. R., RUNCK, A. H. and McCALLUM, L. E.: Observations on autologous previously frozen, deglycerolized, agglomerated, resuspended red cells. I. Effect of storage temperatures. II. Effect of adenine supplementation of glycerolized red cells prior to freezing. *Transfusion*, **7**(2): 105–116, 1967.

VALERI, C. R. and BRODINE, C. E.: Current methods for processing frozen red cells. *Cryobiology*, **5**: 129–135, 1968a.

VALERI, C. R.: Preservation of human red blood cells. *Bull. N. Y. Acad. Med.*, **44**: 3–17, 1968b.

VALERI, C. R. and RUNCK, A. H.: Long term frozen storage of human red blood cells. *Transfusion*, **9**: 5–14, 1969a.

VALERI, C. R., RUNCK, A. H. and BRODINE, C. E.: Recent advances in freeze preservation of red blood cells. *J. Amer. Med. Ass.*, **208**: 489–492, 1969b.

VALERI, C. R. and NATHAN, M. H.: Restoration *in vivo* of erythrocyte adenosine triphosphate, 2, 3-diphosphoglycerate, potassium ion, and sodium ion concentrations, following the transfusion of acid-citrate-dextrose-stored human red blood cells. *J. Laborat. Clin. Med.*, **73**: 722–733, 1969.

VALERI, C. R., SZYMANSKI, I. O. and RUNCK, A. H.: Therapeutic effectiveness of homologous erythrocyte transfusion following frozen storage at −80°C for up to seven years. *Transfusion*, **10**: 102–112, 1970.

VALERI, C. R.: Viability and function of preserved red cells. *New England J. Med.*, **284**: 81–88, 1971.

VINOGRAD-FINKEL, F. R., KISSELE, A. E. and GINZBURG, F. G.: Preservation of blood at ultra-
    low temperatures, The 13th International Congress of Refrigeration, Washington, D.C.,
    1971.

WADA, T., TAKAKU, F., NAKAO, K., NAKAO, M., NAKAO, T. and YOSHIKAWA, H.: Posttransfu-
    sion survival of the red blood cells stored in a medium containing adenine and inosine.
    Proc. Japan. Acad., **36**: 618–623, 1960.

WALLACH, S., ZEMP, J. W., CAVINS, J. A., JENKINS, L. J., JR., BETHEA, M., FRESHETTE, L.,
    HAYNES, L. L. and TULLIS, J. L.: Cation flux and electrolyte composition of frozen-
    deglycerolized blood. *Blood*, **20**: 344–353, 1962.

WEISS, A. J. and BALLINGER, W. F.: The feasibility of storage of intact platelets with appar-
    ent prevention of function. *Ann. Surg.*, **148**: 360–364, 1958.

WERCH, J., GRAY, R. E., HERSH, T. and MELNICK, J. L.: Detection of Australia antigen in
    various fractions of frozen blood. *J. Amer. Med. Ass.*, **218**: 93–94, 1971.

WESSLING, F. C. and BLACKSHEAR, P. L.: The effects of gases on the recovery of human red
    blood cells. *Cryobiology*, **7**: 266–274, 1970.

WESSLING, F. C. and BLACKSHEAR, P. L.: The effects of gases on the recovery of human red
    blood cells. *Cryobiology*, **7**: 265–273, 1971.

WOLSTENHOLME, G. E. W. and O'CONNOR, M. (eds.): The frozen cells, A Ciba Foundation
    Symposium on the Frozen Cell, J. & A. Churchill, London, 1970.

YOSHIKAWA, H. and NAKAO, M.: Nucleotide metabolism and its regulation to functions of pre-
    served human erythrocyte. *Folia Haemat.*, **78**: 248–256, 1962.

ZEMP, J. W. and O'BRIEN, T. G.: *In-vitro* characteristics of glycerolized and frozen human red
    cells. In: Proceedings of the 8th International Congress on Haematology, Vol. 2, pp. 1189,
    1960.

Name Index

Subject Index